A matter of FAT

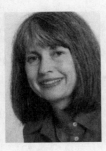

DR ROSEMARY STANTON OAM is one of Australia's best-known nutritionists. Author of many scientific papers on various nutrition and public health topics, 31 books and over 3000 articles for magazines and newspapers, Stanton is a regular presenter on television, a frequent guest on radio programs and a popular lecturer.

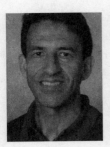

DR ANDREW HILLS is Associate Professor, School of Human Movement Studies, Queensland University of Technology. He has been President of the Australasian Society for the Study of Obesity, is a Fellow of Sports Medicine Australia and is Secretary–Treasurer of the International Council for Physical Activity and Fitness Research.

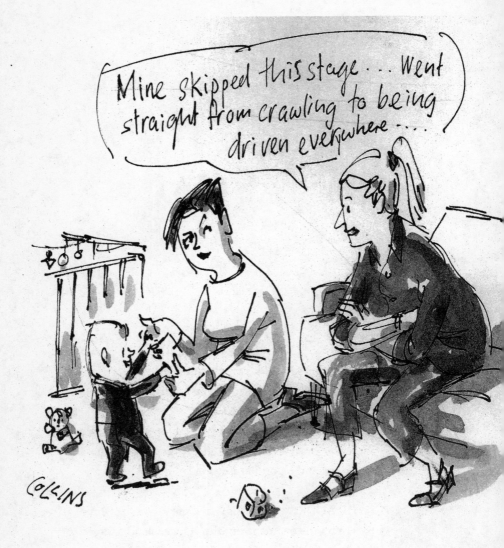

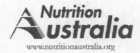

Rosemary Stanton Andrew Hills

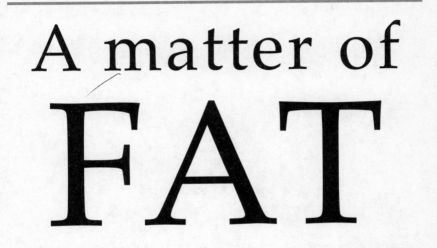

A matter of FAT

Understanding and Overcoming Obesity in Kids

Illustrations by Richard Collins

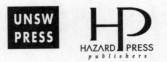

UNSW PRESS

HAZARD PRESS
publishers

A UNSW PRESS BOOK

Published in Australia and the rest of the world except for New Zealand by
University of New South Wales Press Ltd
University of New South Wales
Sydney NSW 2052
AUSTRALIA
www.unswpress.com.au

Published in New Zealand by
Hazard Press
PO Box 2151
Christchurch
www.hazardpress.com

National Library of Australia
Cataloguing-in-Publication entry:

Stanton, Rosemary.
A matter of fat : understanding and overcoming obesity in kids.
Bibliography.
Includes index.
ISBN 0 86840 543 4.

1. Obesity in children. 2. Obesity in children – Prevention.
I. Hills, Andrew P. II. Title.

618.92398

Design Di Quick
Printer Southwood Press

Contents

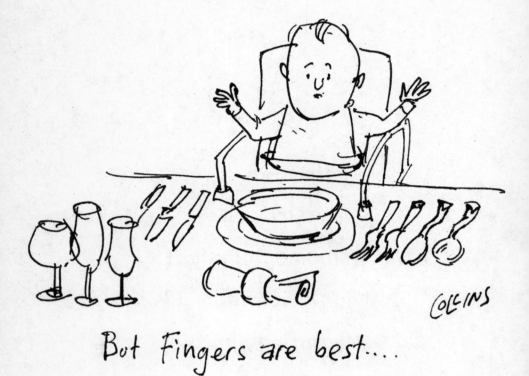

But Fingers are best....

Foreword

In this book, we have tried to answer some common questions about overweight and obesity in children. The simple questions are often the most difficult, but we have found parents want them discussed. How do we know when someone is overweight or obese? What is the normal level of body fat for children during the growing years? What can you do if your child is overweight?

Overweight and obesity are major public health problems throughout the world. With the abundance of food available in places like Australia, the United States and Europe, this might be expected, but excess weight in children is also becoming a major problem throughout Asia and even throughout the third world excess weight is now as great a problem as undernutrition.

Even though overweight and obesity are now so common, the associated problems are often ignored and misinformation abounds. We give the facts about body fat, good eating and healthy activities for children.

We take a good look at the risks, the definitions, at what is normal and at the dual problems of a society obsessed with slimness while people of all ages and both sexes grow steadily fatter.

We don't offer extreme solutions and magic bullets because there aren't any, but we have lots of practical suggestions to help families where one or more members are overweight or obese. We also believe good food is delicious and that there are enjoyable ways to be more active. Our guidelines are practical, enjoyable and based on sound science.

Andrew Hills PhD
Rosemary Stanton OAM PhD

Introduction

As a result of overeating, Templeton grew bigger and fatter than any rat you ever saw. He was gigantic. He was as big as a young woodchuck.

The old sheep spoke to him about his size one day. 'You would live longer,' said the old sheep, 'if you ate less.'

'Who wants to live forever?' sneered the rat. 'I am naturally a heavy eater and I get untold satisfaction from the pleasures of the feast.' He patted his stomach, grinned at the sheep, and crept upstairs to lie down.

EB WHITE, *Charlotte's Web*

Having enough good food to eat is one of life's joys and when what we eat and drink is balanced with what our bodies need, the combination is linked with good health and happiness. But when the balance is tipped so we eat and drink more than what we need, we grow fatter. Too much fat may help keep out the cold and make it easier to float in water, but it has few other advantages.

How common is it?

We have no reliable data from the past, but anecdotally, many people remember a couple of fat children at their school. They were noticeable because there were so few of them. That's not the case these days. There are many more fat kids around and we have the numbers to prove it.

The prevalence of excess weight depends on the population studied and the way overweight and obesity are defined. For adults, the standard definition is usually based on body mass index or BMI. (We discuss this in Chapter 3.) For children, an allowance is also made for the child's age. Using these criteria, in Australia, 64% of men, 47% of women and just over 20% of 2 to 18-year-olds are overweight or obese. In some age groups, the problem is even greater.

The figures below, based on an Australian National Nutrition Survey in 1995, give us an idea of how the problem is distributed over childhood and between the sexes:*

	% OVERWEIGHT OR OBESE	
AGE (YEARS)	BOYS	GIRLS
2–3	28	23
4–7	19	24
8–11	18	32
12–15	29	24
16–18	32	27

* Magarey, AM, Daniels, LA and Boulton, TJ., *Medical Journal of Australia*, 2001; 174(11): 561–4.

Since then, studies in Victorian primary school children have reported that 12.5% of 5 to 6-year-olds are overweight and another 7.5% are obese (a total of 20%). By ages 10–12, 13% are overweight and 10.5% are obese. A recent New South Wales Schools Fitness and Physical Activity Study found 22% of primary school children were overweight or obese.

Obesity is now the biggest public health problem of our time. It's so common and so worrying that some describe it as an epidemic. In the 10 years between 1985 and 1995, overweight and obesity in Australian children increased dramatically. During this period, the number of overweight 7–15 year-olds almost doubled and those classified as obese more than tripled. Similar problems have also occurred in many other countries throughout the world.

What is obesity?

We need to distinguish between *overweight* and *obesity*. Overweight refers to an increase in body weight, usually defined in relation to height, above a standard considered as optimal for health. Overweight easily leads to obesity, defined as an excessive proportion of body fat. Kids come in all shapes and sizes and you can't always tell the difference between overweight and obesity just by looking at a child. We also have different ideas of what is too fat, usually based on cultural and family perceptions, so an official assessment is useful to decide if a problem exists. One method of assessing obesity in children uses a formula that includes calculating BMI from height and weight as well as measuring waist and skinfold thickness.

Why are so many children overweight or obese? The simple answer is that children have grown fatter as a result of doing less physical activity while consuming as much, or more energy from food and drinks. In the past, most kids were active around the house and walked to school or the shops. They also spent a lot of time outside, built cubby houses, explored their neighbourhood, made and raced billycarts and played games such as backyard cricket. However, in 1985, as many as 30% of Australian children aged between 9 and 15 failed to meet the minimum standard for heart–lung fitness. By the mid-90s this had risen to 60%.

Obesity involves a complex mix of factors, including physiology, biochemistry, metabolism, anatomy, psychology and social aspects. This makes it difficult to come up with a simple definition, but in all cases of obesity, there is an increase in body fat and body weight.

Defining obesity in children and adolescents is complicated because their body fat can vary from year to year and is also related to their level of sexual development. However, both boys and girls who are obese have high levels of body fat. This can be measured by trained experts. Using good measuring techniques, an acceptable level of body fat before puberty is 17–18% of total body weight. By age 18, this changes and the usual acceptable level of body fat is 15–18% for boys and 20–25% for girls.

Some definitions of childhood obesity rate a child's height and weight compared with other children of the same age and sex. Children in the top 5% of weight for height and age (often referred to as being above the 95th percentile) are defined as obese. Others restrict the definition to the top 3% of weight for height and age. Such definitions may be useful for comparing children within a population but don't necessarily reflect desirable weights for an individual child.

Does obesity matter?

Yes! Obesity is more common today than ever before and is occurring at much younger ages throughout the world. In poorer countries, overweight and obese rich children co-exist with those who are hungry and homeless. This paradox can be explained by two reasons: many rich people have the money to buy highly processed foods (often a status symbol) and may engage in less physical activity than their poorer counterparts. Poor people, on the other hand, often lack the resources to make wise food choices. The point to remember is that obesity matters wherever it occurs because it can contribute to physical and social problems in children and adolescents.

Physical problems

- accelerated growth and early physical maturity
- insulin resistance and type 2 diabetes*
- asthma
- high blood fats
- high blood pressure
- orthopaedic problems
- breathing difficulties, including sleep apnoea

13

*Insulin normally takes glucose out of the blood into the cells where it can be used for energy. Insulin resistance occurs when a layer of fat builds up in the membrane around each cell and impedes the action of insulin. Glucose then builds up in the blood and the body tries to compensate by producing more insulin. This leads to type 2 diabetes where blood glucose and insulin levels are high, while the cells are denied their normal supply of energy. Children and most adults who develop type 2 diabetes are obese.

Obese children have a 25–50% chance of becoming obese adults and this can increase to about 80% for obese adolescents. Overweight or obese adults then have a greatly increased risk of type 2 diabetes, coronary heart disease, high blood pressure, many types of cancer and more problems with backs, feet and joints.

The incidence of type 2 diabetes is particularly worrying. In adults, this serious health problem greatly increases the risk of coronary heart disease, high blood pressure, kidney problems and blindness. Once seen only in those over 50, type 2 diabetes is now occurring in obese adolescents and children as young as 10 years of age.

Psycho-social problems

- poor body image and low self-confidence
- poor daytime concentration resulting from sleep apnoea
- bullying and teasing from other children
- behavioural problems

As well as the medical consequences of obesity, some hurtful people make fun of fat kids (and adults), making them a prime target for many social and emotional problems. Even among some very young children, there are strong feelings against the overweight body. When a group of pre-school children was asked to rate pictures of people of varying size and shape, its members consistently rated fat children as less likeable than children with physical handicaps.

If obese children have problems making friends, they may develop a lack of self-confidence, as well as a dislike or even feelings of disgust towards their bodies. Some obese children may become withdrawn, resent being around normal-weight children and shy away from physical activity.

With so many potential problems to the individual as well as future health care costs to society leading on from obesity in childhood, it's obvious we need to prevent it.

Can anything be done?

Yes! Although there is a common perception that all overweight children will end up as obese adults, it is certainly not inevitable that fat children will stay fat and many achieve and maintain normal weight. However, it is likely that a large percentage of overweight and obese children will have problems with excess weight throughout their lives — which is why we recommend taking action.

As soon as children learn to toddle, they are keen to walk and then to run around. However, with our society's emphasis on speed and efficiency, we often force toddlers into a pram or stroller to make our own lives easier, sometimes silencing their protests by giving them something to eat while we strap them in. This deprives these children of their natural instinct to walk and soon the sitting habit becomes so entrenched that they expect to sit and be pushed around or carried.

This is the way bad habits develop easily and early, against the natural inclination of our children towards movement. Sitting in front of a television is another bad habit we teach our children to make life easier for ourselves. After all, playing more actively creates more mess and needs greater supervision when children are little. In fact, active playing when young leads to better habits of being able to play actively later. And going outside to play rather than sitting watching television or playing computer games is a great way to help prevent obesity.

Some people think overweight children will grow out of their 'puppy fat'. Sadly, puppy fat tends to become a faithful hound and obesity in children rarely corrects itself spontaneously. Some direct intervention is vital.

Physical activity

If any of us are asked to do something we don't like or can't do, we feel uncomfortable and are likely to avoid repeating such bad experiences, so we need to be patient with our expectations for children and tolerant of those who may be less skilful at sport.

Some obese children hate physical activity and lack any motivation to participate in it. This often means they are left out of games and sports, perpetuating a vicious cycle of lack of activity, greater levels of fatness and continued lack of movement. The cycle needs to be broken. Kids need to discover that physical activity can be fun but it's worth starting a new regime gently. No one likes to be a failure, irrespective of body size, so strategies for changing behaviour should include those that are not stressful so the child can cope and have some success. To start with, this may be a few minutes of walking, riding a bike, swimming or playing some sport the child likes, extending the time as the child becomes fitter. Chapter 6 gives strategies for increasing physical activity for children of all ages, from infants to young adults.

Nutrition

Good nutrition is important from the time of conception. For all children, irrespective of their size, healthy food should be part of their daily lives. There is no magic age to start good eating and better activity patterns — the earlier the better. But don't despair if your child is already overweight. It is possible to gradually change unhealthy eating habits without too much stress, especially if you keep away from diets. Good eating habits for children involve healthier meals and snacks — *not* **restrictive** dieting. See Chapter 5 for suggestions for nutritious and delicious menus for children.

While children are growing, it is best to try to alter body composition and keep weight steady rather than aiming for actual weight-loss. If children adopt appropriate new eating and exercise patterns and stay the same weight while they grow in height, they will become slimmer. Even if it takes one or more years for a child to gradually slim down, once he or she is no longer obese, the chance of becoming an obese adult decreases.

What if it's in the genes?

Just because your family has a history of overweight and obesity doesn't mean you can't do anything about it. The old saying *prevention is better than cure* definitely applies to obesity. It is easier to teach children skills to maximise good health rather than trying to change established bad habits later in life. To prevent obesity, we need to establish good habits *before* there are signs of excess weight. This is important for everyone, but giving young children healthy foods and plenty of physical activity as early as possible is especially vital for those children at high risk of obesity because their parents or other family members are obese.

There is a strong association between obesity in children and their parents' weight. The good news is that treating a child's obesity with changes in eating and exercise habits can benefit the whole family.

What if my child is already obese?

For parents with children who are already obese and may not like healthy foods or walking, don't despair — there *are* effective ways to help or at least prevent them becoming fatter. Chapters 5 and 6 discuss strategies.

An individual approach

Obese children have some common traits, but every child has a distinct personality and health status, as well as individual eating and activity habits. Failing to understand individual differences, especially in physical growth and development, can lead to a generalised approach to treating obesity that is unlikely to be effective for a particular child. A 'generic' approach to obesity and failing to cater for individual needs may be why treating childhood obesity has had poor outcomes in the past.

Essentially, there are three approaches to treating weight control, using the principles of energy balance:

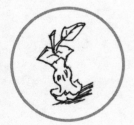

1 to be more physically active while making no change to what you eat and drink;

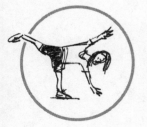

2 to consume fewer kilojoules in food and drinks and make no change to physical activity;

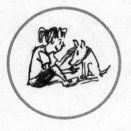

3 a combination of consuming fewer kilojoules and increasing physical activity.

The bigger picture

Some pessimists believe it is impossible to do anything about childhood obesity. However, assessing BMI, waist circumferences and skinfold thickness can help identify children who may be at high risk of later obesity so preventive measures can start early. Governments, parents, teachers and children can all play a role in improving children's health and body composition. We also need to lobby for changes in our eating and exercise environment to make it easier. When cigarette advertising and smoking in the workplace and many public areas were phased out, it made it much easier for people to change their smoking habits. By tackling the problem effectively, we can reduce a major public health problem. The greatest challenge is to put into place effective strategies to change the 'obesogenic environment' in which we live. We discuss this in Chapter 7.

1

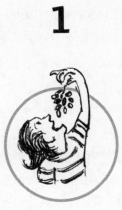

Understanding
obesity

To help your children get into better shape, it's important to understand why they are affected by obesity. Appreciating the issues involved will help in finding a solution (or solutions). Essentially, the main causes are:

- **MEDICAL**

    Endocrine (gland) problems are extremely rare, but if in doubt, seek further medical investigation. There is also a possible link between poor growth in the uterus and later obesity.

- **A GENETIC PREDISPOSITION**

    There is still confusion over the relative contribution genes make to obesity. Although genes undoubtedly play a role in the degree of weight gained, more research is currently being carried out to discover why. Although there has been an increase in obesity over the last few years, there have been no genetic changes during this period.

- **DIET**

    Recent surveys show that children and adolescents are eating more than they used to and the increase is enough to explain the higher incidence of overweight and obesity. Consuming too many high-energy foods and drinks is a major factor.

- **PHYSICAL INACTIVITY**

  The fall in physical activity in the home, at school and during leisure times are important contributors to excess body fat. The fatter a child becomes, the greater the tendency not to exercise because physical activity becomes uncomfortable and potentially embarrassing.

- **PSYCHO-SOCIAL FACTORS**

  Personality traits, depression, family size, socio-economic status, motivation and eating disorders can be relevant to the development and maintenance of obesity.

As we can see, there is no mystery to the major factors involved in obesity. They include poor eating habits and low levels of physical activity superimposed on a genetic tendency to gain weight. All excess weight is a result of an energy imbalance between the kilojoules of energy coming into the body and those we expend. However, this simple explanation ignores the complex reasons why imbalances occur. We know that anyone who continues to eat more than the body needs for growth and physical activity will gain body fat, but not everyone who leads a 'couch potato' lifestyle becomes obese.

A genetic predisposition

Obesity often runs in families and while this may reflect a family's eating and exercise habits, genetic factors are also important. The relative contributions made to obesity by genes and environmental factors are not yet known, but we know both are involved.

Studies of identical twins demonstrate the role of genes. The idea that some people can eat as much as they like and never gain a gram is a myth. When people are overfed (taking account of their usual requirements, age, size, sex and other relevant factors), they *all* gain weight. But some gain more than others. Studies in which twins are overfed show each pair of twins gains a remarkably similar amount of extra weight. However, when compared with other pairs, the amount of weight they gain will be different. Thus, with the same degree of overfeeding, one pair may gain 3 kg while another pair may gain 6 kg.

We also know that some babies are genetically programmed to move more than others from birth onwards and possibly even before birth. These children may escape the consequences of bad eating habits because they move more, both at play, during sport and even when apparently sitting still. Genes appear to be responsible for inbuilt 'fidget' activity, which can burn up many kilojoules a day. Just as genes can make some people better at some kinds of sport, they also influence other factors that affect body weight, such as height, frame size, body shape and the proportion of different muscle fibres.

Lots of research studies are underway, but even before all their results are published, we can safely say that a proportion of the population has a genetic predisposition to obesity and thus finds it more difficult to maintain a constant body weight in an environment that supplies constant encouragement to eat and drink more while minimising physical activity. Some people seem to have inherited genes that allow them better inbuilt balance between what they eat and how much energy they expend.

THE MYTH OF 'GLANDS'

Contrary to popular belief, glands are almost never a reason for obesity. Malfunctioning of the thyroid gland can alter metabolic rate, but studies show that those who are obese do not suffer from low metabolism. Any abnormalities in thyroid function can easily be normalised with appropriate medications.

During pregnancy

Some factors favouring easy weight gain may also occur due to environmental factors before birth. There is some evidence that, in some cases, obesity later in life may have its origins in the womb. Excessive weight gain during pregnancy may be a factor, but perversely, too little weight gain during pregnancy may also be a problem. If a pregnant woman is undernourished, her child may have difficulty regulating the way the body uses fats and sugars later in life.

Professor David Barker from Hertfordshire has done some amazing detective work in the United Kingdom. According to what has become known as 'the Barker hypothesis', women who do not gain enough weight during pregnancy put their infants at significant health risk of problems many years later. Barker and his co-workers traced people from their birth records and found a relationship between low birth weight and small placental weight and an impaired ability to handle blood glucose 60 years later. These small babies (and the small placentas that were also a feature of their births) were poorly nourished during pregnancy.

Barker's hypothesis fits with the Dutch Hunger Winter study that looked at pregnant women who endured a near-starvation diet in Nazi-occupied Holland between December 1944 and April 1945. Women who had been denied adequate food in the last trimester of pregnancy produced babies who were lighter, shorter and had a smaller head circumference and less placental area. Follow-up studies at 19 years of age showed that these young people had a greater incidence of obesity and a surprisingly high incidence of type 2 diabetes. By age 50, they had increased levels of insulin in the blood and high levels of blood glucose. Those who had become overweight had the worst levels and more males than females were adversely affected.

Studies from the Department of Obstetrics and Gynaecology at Adelaide University have also found that maternal diet during critical stages of pregnancy affects the development of the baby and programs its growth and potential to develop obesity later in life. These and other studies show that too little weight gain due to poor nutrition during pregnancy may be related to future obesity.

On the other hand, there are also potential problems if women gain excessive amounts of weight during each pregnancy. Without any increase in the kilojoules they consume, some women with babies weighing 3.5 kg can also increase their own body fat by 4 kg or more during pregnancy. It appears that a pregnant woman needs to eat enough nutrients for herself and her baby, but she does not need to double her kilojoule intake by 'eating for two'. Pregnancy is not a time to restrict nutrients but eating whenever and whatever you feel like is also not ideal for baby or mother. The way to achieve balance in supplying enough for the baby, but not too much excess for the mother, may be for pregnant women to eat ample quantities of good food but restrict foods of low nutritional value. The Weight Watchers organisation reports that most of their members claim their weight problems developed during pregnancy. And the more pregnancies they undergo, the greater their weight problems.

Diet

What we eat and drink has a major influence on health. You don't have to be a rocket scientist to realise that the current easy-to-eat, high-fat, high-sugar, high-kilojoule diet has a major effect on body weight. The *way* we eat is also important and also influences *what* we eat.

Eating habits

The eating habits that last most people throughout life are established in infancy. The most important lesson to teach children may be to eat when they are hungry and stop when they have had enough. Sadly, we often ruin babies' natural appetite control by encouraging them to drink a defined quantity of infant formula, instead of letting them suck from the breast at will. There is good evidence that breast feeding without adding any other foods for the first 6 months of life helps reduce the incidence of excess weight. It's also important not to praise children for finishing whatever we give them to eat.

When so many commonly available and widely advertised foods contribute many kilojoules from their high content of fat, sugar or both, it is remarkably easy to eat more than you need. No one food or drink is responsible for obesity — it is the total kilojoule level of the diet and whether it balances with what the body needs that counts. It's worth remembering that it is almost impossible to over-consume foods such as fruits, vegetables or wholegrain products because their fibre is filling.

How much do we eat?

There are regular surveys to find out what people are eating but it's a difficult thing to measure, partly because the food supply is now so complex. In the 1960s, a country like Australia had 600–800 different foods available at various times of the year and most people's diets were relatively constant. The average Australian supermarket now stocks around 12–15,000 items while many in the United States may have 4 to 10 times that number.

Most people under-report what they eat and drink. If asked to keep specific records of their food consumption, most people change their usual pattern and many lose weight. Because fat and sugar have had bad publicity, many people specifically under-report their intake. This is not always deliberate, but it makes it difficult to estimate how much children and adults are eating. However, studies using the same methodology clearly show that children consumed many more kilojoules in the mid 1990s compared with the mid 80s. Comprehensive data since then is not yet available, but sales data for snack foods and fast foods would indicate that overall kilojoule intake continues to climb. Supermarkets currently stock 1750 different snack foods.

Snacking

In many families, regular meals eaten together at a table have been replaced by a pattern of individual snacks. Children often take responsibility for their own meals and snacks and if they don't have adequate skills to prepare or cook foods, their diets may suffer as a result.

Convenience foods

A rushed lifestyle — whether real or perceived — makes a strong indirect contribution to obesity. How many of us eat a range of packaged and highly processed foods in favour of foods prepared at home from fresh ingredients?

The theory is that convenience foods are a quick, no-fuss, acceptable alternative to creating a meal from scratch. Food companies use time-poor concepts to push convenience and fast foods. Marketing and advertising have helped convince many people to choose this path. Many of these foods are of dubious nutritional value, with higher levels of fat, salt and sugar and less dietary fibre than similar foods prepared at home from scratch. Some families ignore such potential problems for the sake of convenience. Others simply don't know how to prepare fast healthier meals from basic fresh ingredients. Some sellers of convenience foods play on this by implying that cooking is time-consuming and difficult.

Genuine problems with time may involve domestic arrangements where women work outside the home but are also responsible for shopping and preparing food. It's not so much that many women dread cooking, but more the burden of having to take responsibility for deciding what the family will eat and having the relevant ingredients on hand. This situation is changing gradually and more men are now helping with domestic chores. However, the majority of men and children have few cooking skills and women still take the lion's share of the food load.

Junk food

We are faced with an amazing array of high energy foods and drinks. Consequently, we have learned to eat and drink whether we are hungry or not. Advertising directed at children is remarkably effective in altering their diet and generates strong peer pressure to include particular branded foods and drinks.

Foods also change and many people are unaware of this. For example, who would have guessed that the average hamburger in the 1970s had about half the fat level of the modern fast food burgers or that potato crisps are now sold in 50 g or 100 g packets compared with individual 28 g servings 30 years ago?

Fat intake is also increasing as people consume more processed snack foods and eat out more often. Marketing surveys show one-third of the food budget in Australia is spent on foods prepared away from home and restaurant and take-away foods are much fattier than home-cooked meals.

Physical activity

Safety

As cities become more crowded, parents have concerns for the safety of their children playing in the neighbourhood and getting themselves to school. This can mean that parents no longer allow their children to walk or cycle to school. Activities such as playing in the bush or going off on bicycles may also be seen as unsafe. In many families, parents are not home after school and some set rules that children must stay inside the home rather than going out to play.

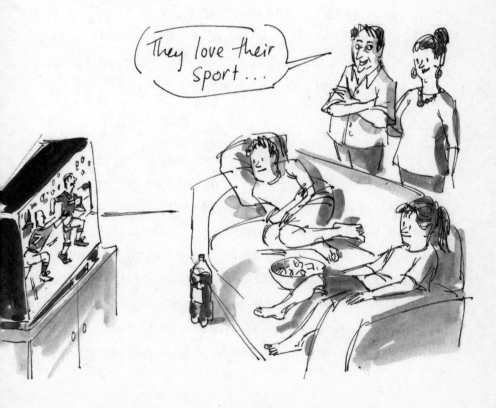

There is a strong link between perceptions of safety and television. For some parents, television becomes almost a substitute 'safe' babysitter. Many studies show that obesity is directly related to time spent watching television. For many children and adolescents, the only daily activity that occupies more time than television, computers and video games is sleep. Most children also eat while watching television — and advertising provides constant reminders to do so. Although safety is a legitimate concern, a culture of fear can easily become an impediment to children's activity and health, restricting opportunies for physical activity.

Houses have also generally become larger but backyards have shrunk. Some backyards are designed for entertaining rather than being free space for playing and few people now have space for children to play active games. The high value of vacant land has also decreased available recreation space in many localities. Safety is an associated concern, particularly for parents of young children.

The time factor

Time constraints also have adverse effects on our health. Few people think they have time to walk, even for short distances. Where there is a lack of public transport greater reliance is placed on private cars to take kids to school. Again, safety is a legitimate concern, but it can be a stumbling block to children's activity and a factor in obesity. Statistics also show that being a passenger in a car presents a greater danger than walking to school, although few parents consider this as they drive kids everywhere.

Labour-saving devices

As a society, we condone low levels of physical activity by always looking for opportunities to minimise energy expenditure. We teach children habits that emphasise labour saving with such devices as remote controls, push-button windows, lifts, car parks under buildings, drive-through fast food outlets and even automatic central controls for appliances. One gadget is being developed whereby a centralised control panel will turn on appliances throughout the home, open the curtains and even unlatch the front door for approved visitors (viewed on a screen) to enter the house. Somewhat ironically, the device will be implanted into the door of the fridge!

Day-to-day movement

We now have a society in which the total level of activity, including day-to-day habitual movement plus all forms of exercise, including walking and playing sport, is less than the habitual movement of previous generations. A combination of low levels of physical activity and a high intake of fatty or sugary foods make it particularly easy for children to take in more energy than they expend. Similar factors have caused obesity in every country where they have become the norm. The United States, Canada, Australia and the United Kingdom were the first examples, but as Asian, European and Middle Eastern countries adopt similar lifestyles, their populations too are showing rapid increases in obesity.

Some children naturally move so much during play and when apparently sitting still that they burn up lots of energy. Some of these children may appear to be able to eat a lot —

including junk food — without gaining weight. However, junk foods can still cause a build-up of fat in the arteries and may displace other more nutritious foods.

Sedentary habits

Physical activity is essential for children's normal growth and development and children need the opportunity to develop the necessary motor skills to participate in physical activity from an early age. More active pursuits tend to suffer as a result of so much time in sedentary activities such as watching television or videos and playing computer games. The highly competitive atmosphere surrounding some sports also means many children who do not excel at sport drop out early. The popularity of spectator sports also means that most people sit and watch a small number being active. This is quite different from a personal commitment to physical activity.

Psycho-social factors

Sleep apnoea

Overweight children can suffer from sleep apnoea, a condition that is caused when the throat muscles relax during sleep and obstruct the air flow, causing the sleeper to wake. If these children do not get a good night's sleep as a result, they may doze off frequently during the day and find it difficult to pay attention in school. This can have adverse effects on their studies and also leads to other more alert children making fun of them. The general lack of energy and tiredness that arises from sleep apnoea thus has physical and psychological effects.

Peer pressure

Bullying and teasing can make obesity worse, as was witnessed one afternoon. An overweight child walking home from school was being teased by his friends who were calling him 'Fatty', pushing him and then running so he couldn't catch them. Obviously sick of it all, he retreated into a small shop and emerged about 10 minutes later to walk home alone, eating a large packet of crisps and an iceblock.

Even among very young children, the societal perception of thinness and overweight can reinforce the prejudice against obesity and inadvertently contribute to it. For example, young girls and boys who are dissatisfied with their size and shape can become preoccupied with their weight. Often, healthy eating is confused with dieting.

The latest diet can bring great profits for magazines and the authors of diet books. These diets vary dramatically. Depending on the fad of the moment, they may be high or low in fat, protein or carbohydrate. Some impose strict rules about what you can eat and drink. Others are designed to sell supplements, powders, drinks or some snack that is intended to replace meals. Most claim to be *the* way to lose weight quickly and easily. Almost any diet will work in the short term, but there's little evidence that most are of long-term benefit in maintaining weight-loss and their ability to induce poor body image and loss of self-confidence makes them doubly dangerous, especially for children.

However, not all fat children are friendless or unhealthy. Many cope well with excess weight, maintaining a cheerful

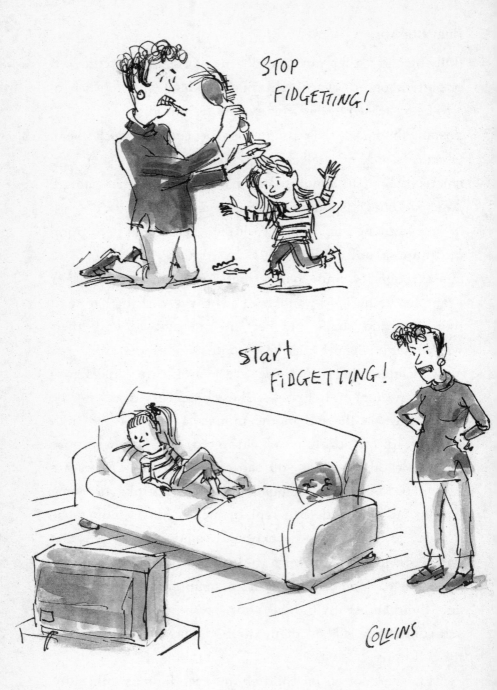

disposition and taking part happily in all activities at school and with their friends. It's important to consider each child as an individual who may cope well or have problems, whatever their size.

The power of advertising

Weight disorders, including obesity, can be the result of the influence of the media. Television programs and advertisements emphasise lean, tall, 'beautiful' people. Most women and girls shown are slim and males are usually muscular. Few people fit such idealised images. Models are usually chosen *because* they are different from the norm. Sadly, a paradox then occurs with many normal-sized teenagers beginning to think their body size and shape are wrong. Some may diet excessively or develop serious eating and weight disorders such as anorexia nervosa, bulimia or obesity.

There is evidence that dieting itself can lead many teenage girls down the path to obesity. After following a strict diet, some girls then more than make up for their dieting by binge-eating the formerly forbidden foods. Feeling guilty for their indulgence, they then start another diet, which usually has a similar outcome. The habit of dieting and binge-eating can easily become entrenched, along with feelings of loss of control and low self-confidence.

2

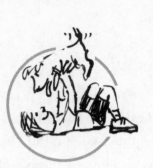

What is normal?

Obesity means an abnormal amount of body weight is composed of fat. Beyond this simple definition there are no widely accepted ways of classifying obesity. Weight, on its own, does not necessarily indicate fat content. Some people have large skeletal frames and well-developed muscles and may be heavy, but fit and not over-fat. Some children may also weigh more than others of the same age because they are physically more mature.

To decide whether your child does have a problem with overweight or obesity, it's useful to know something about the process of growth and development. Hopefully, the more we know and understand about the wide variability in size, shape, body composition and individual growth patterns of our children, the more tolerant we will be of difference as well as helping our children and adolescents cope better with the dramatic changes that occur.

The most significant physical changes from childhood to adulthood are in height, weight, body composition and body proportions. To understand the normal physical changes during the growing years, let's look at the terms commonly used. The terms *growth* and *development* are often used interchangeably, although technically they are different.

Growth refers to an increase in physical size of the body or any of its component parts. Individual body parts do not grow at the same rate. Good examples of growth are the obvious changes in height and weight that occur during childhood. Less obvious examples include repair of tissues in skin, muscle or bone after injury. If children break a bone, the tissue grows and regenerates much better than will occur in adults. The capacity

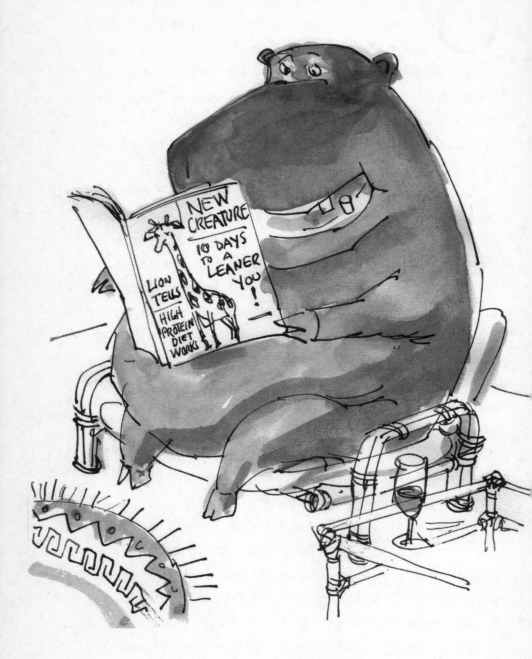

for tissues to 'bounce back' after damage decreases as we age.

Development refers to any improvement in skill or bodily function and includes a child's ability in more advanced motor skills. Children move progressively from reflex movements that are uncoordinated to skills such as walking and running that take lots of control.

There are no definite rules to identify the boundaries between these stages because changes in growth and development for each individual are continuous and not confined to a distinct age. Growth and development are not necessarily smooth and homogeneous and, except for identical twins, no two people are alike. However, there are particular features of growth and development that are considered normal for the specific stages of infancy, childhood and adolescence.

There are many normal differences in growth and development between boys and girls. In boys, growth occurs over a longer time period and physical dimensions, including height, may continue to change into their mid-twenties. Tissues such as muscle and bone may continue growing for even longer.

Rate of growth

The growth process for any individual child resembles that of all children up to a point, but each child has a unique timetable and individual differences occur at all stages of growth and development. For this reason, mean or average values for height and weight should be used only as a rough guide, although we can get some idea of health status by noting whether a child's height and weight are consistent with other children of the same sex and age. These are more important indicators of appropriate growth for a child than whether he or she is tall or short.

In general, girls are more physically advanced than boys of the same age. Even at birth, a girl's body is more mature and the average baby girl is about 4 weeks more skeletally mature than the average newborn boy. Girls also grow up faster, reach puberty earlier and consequently finish their growth at an earlier age than boys.

Changes in height and weight can also be described in terms of speed or velocity — for example, in centimetres of growth or increase in kilograms per year. The most rapid growth in height occurs immediately after birth in the first year of life, then the speed of growth declines throughout childhood. Babies and young children are normally rounded, with their fat more pronounced because of their relatively large trunk and short limbs. Except for the first year of life, children grow more rapidly in height than in weight. During much of the primary school years, children's arms and legs grow fast and some children appear to be 'all arms and legs'. As the body lengthens through the early school years, children become leaner. At about 7 years of age, most girls and some boys accumulate a bit more fat and may look slightly chubbier. Some become self-conscious about this.

A second and dramatic increase occurs at puberty when children reach their period of peak height and weight velocity. This is normally when most young people grow the most (in terms of centimetres or kilograms) in a one-year period.

The rate of growth differs at various stages. By 4–5 years of age, yearly growth is about a quarter of that seen during the first year of life. Growth rate continues to decline until puberty, with little difference between boys and girls throughout childhood. Children also pass through the accelerated phase of growth associated with adolescence at different chronological ages, although they tend to follow a similar pattern or sequence.

Most girls have achieved a high proportion of their overall height by the onset of menstruation (menarche) and the average girl does not grow more than 5–6 cm after her periods begin. The timing of the adolescent growth spurt influences adult height, although the sooner a child enters his or her adolescent growth phase, the earlier they tend to stop growing.

From puberty onwards, distinct male and female physical characteristics become obvious. These differences are due to the influence of hormones, which encourage the growth of particular tissues. Testosterone causes boys' shoulders to widen and their muscle mass to increase. In girls, oestrogen causes redistribution and more rounded fat deposits and is responsible for the widening of the pelvis at the expense of the shoulders.

The stimulus that causes early or delayed growth affects all bodily dimensions. Children who reach puberty early are more likely to be slightly shorter as adults than those who enter this phase later. This is a well-known phenomenon and is logical in that a longer growing period favours growth of longer limbs and greater height.

Changes in body proportions

As well as an increase in the length of the total body and its component parts, growth also involves changes in body proportions. The body of a newborn baby is proportioned differently from that of an adult. In infancy, the size of the head and body (technically, the trunk) dominate the body compared with arms and legs. A baby's head is 22% (almost a quarter) of its length whereas an adult's head is about 13% of total height. Growth changes in the head are similar for boys and girls although the head size of the average boy is slightly larger at all ages. The relative proportion of the length of arms and legs also changes dramatically. At birth, a baby's legs are about three-eighths of the body length. By adulthood, the legs are approximately half the total height.

All parts of the body do not reach mature proportions at the same time, but by mid adolescence, the body has generally assumed its mature proportions. The changes in the proportions of the body are dramatic: from birth to maturity the head doubles in size, the trunk increases in length three times, the arms are four times and the legs approximately five times longer.

During childhood and until puberty, growth of the head is slow, growth of the trunk is intermediate and growth of limbs is more rapid. Even though different parts of the body grow and reach a mature size and shape at different times, on the whole, growth is steady and continuous.

Head

The skull, brain and facial features reach maturity in growth and development before other organs and before the general features of the trunk and limbs mature. Babies are born with a disproportionately large head, which then grows less after birth than most other parts of the body. At first, the cranial vault is dominant and facial features occupy a small area and appear compressed. A child's head is also broader in relation to length than an adult's. The width of the skull reaches its maximum at about three years of age but continues to lengthen until 17–18 years. Boys and girls have similar growth changes, but boys have a slightly larger head at all ages.

The cranium completes its growth early, making the top and back of the head appear too large for the face. Facial features change as the shape of the head changes and undergo the most pronounced changes during the growing years. The small 'pug' nose of a baby stays small in the early years, grows rapidly between 5 and 10 years of age and generally reaches its mature size by about 14 years of age.

Trunk

At about 6 months of age, the trunk is twice as long and twice as wide as at birth. By adult size, the trunk will have trebled in length from birth. Babies have little discernible neck and their head appears to almost sit on their shoulders, while the trunk is somewhat cylindrical in shape. For the first 4–5 years of life, a child's trunk tends to be a bit sack-like with a protruding abdomen, no apparent waistline, sloping shoulders and a rounded chest.

As a result of the disproportionate size of the head, an infant looks decidedly top heavy. During later childhood, the trunk lengthens and its stockiness decreases, the abdomen flattens and a distinct waistline appears. The shape of the trunk in adults is influenced by the age of sexual maturation, but regardless of their stage of maturation, girls' hips grow larger at the expense of their shoulders while the opposite growth pattern occurs in boys.

Arms and legs

At birth, legs appear proportionately too short, arms too long and hands and feet too small. The legs of a newborn baby are short and don't fully extend at the knees. Initially, infants' arms grow faster than their legs and by 8 years of age, arms are nearly 50% longer than they were at age 2. A relative lack of muscle development and little definition of muscle gives children's arms a linear look.

An expert can guess a child's developmental age from physical characteristics, including the proportionality of the body. The proportions and shape of the body (physique) can also determine how suitable and successful the child may be in various competitive sporting activities. However, it is important not to rate success only on whether a child is likely to win gold medals in some sport. Ideally, we should help all children find sports they enjoy, whether or not they will excel at them.

Physical features

Pre-school

Between 2 and 5 years of age:

- head and trunk are large in comparison with extremities, especially legs;

- the large cranial vault at the back of the head is dominant;

- facial features are less developed (many children have a high forehead and 'pug' nose);

- the lower jaw (mandible) is withdrawn and is less prominent than the upper jaw (maxilla);

- the neck is usually short;

- the trunk is relatively large and cylindrical, with a protruding tummy;

- the spinal column is relatively straight and upright;

- arms and legs are not well developed and knock knees are common.

School age

Shortly after 5 years of age, a child's external appearance begins to change. The changes do not occur uniformly and some children appear to move awkwardly as different body parts grow at different times, contrasting with the more stable size and shape in 2–5 year-olds. General changes from age 5 to puberty:

- leaner and more linear bodies;

- arms and legs grow at a faster rate;

- muscle contours become more obvious as body fat decreases;

- the trunk lags in development as limbs grow and the protruding abdomen disappears, with the trunk becoming less cylindrical and a waist appearing;

- facial features catch up and the forehead and the back of the head are less dominant;

- the neck becomes more pronounced and lengthens;

- the natural curvatures of the spine can be seen.

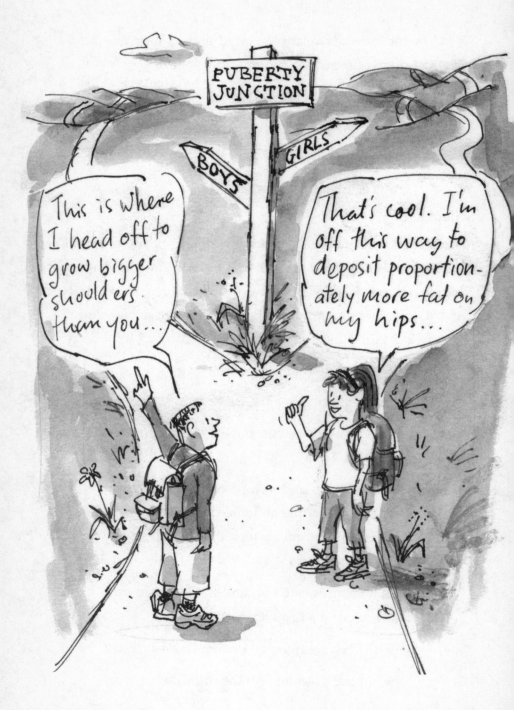

Adolescence

From puberty onwards, distinct male and female physical characteristics become obvious. In girls, the pelvis widens at the expense of the shoulders. In boys, the opposite occurs. Girls also deposit more body fat than boys, who have greater increases in their skeletal muscle.

Sex differences

In general, girls are more physically advanced than boys of the same age. Even at birth, a girl's body is more mature and the average baby girl is about four weeks more skeletally mature than the average newborn boy. Girls also grow up faster, reach puberty earlier and consequently finish their growth at an earlier age than boys.

Some differences between boys and girls depend on their different body shapes, and society's stereotyping also influences the opportunities for boys or girls to be involved in some physical activities. During the pre-pubertal years, there are more physical similarities between boys and girls than there are differences and boys and girls appear to have similar capabilities in physical activity — if given the same opportunities.

Different physical characteristics may influence children's suitability for some activities. When fully grown, the average girl is smaller and has different body proportions, with shorter arms and legs, a longer trunk and a broader pelvis than boys. In some girls, the angle at the hip between the thighbone and pelvis can limit or interfere with the mechanics of running.

Lower levels of haemoglobin — the iron-rich pigment that carries oxygen — can limit the aerobic capacity of some adolescent girls. Many girls also have less muscular strength than boys, partly because they may not use their muscles as much, but also because of basic physiological differences. It is also normal for girls to have higher levels of body fat, and this may limit performance levels in some elite sports.

The greatest differences between girls and boys occur after puberty, due to the influence of testosterone and oestrogen. Both these natural steroid hormones encourage the growth of particular tissues, so some major differences in physique between boys and girls are under hormonal control. Testosterone causes boys' shoulders to widen and their muscle mass to increase. In girls, oestrogen causes redistribution and more rounded fat deposits and is responsible for the widening of the pelvis. Sex hormones are also largely responsible for increasing physiological differences between males and females. Compared with women, men have larger lungs and a bigger heart, a higher resting heart rate and higher systolic blood pressure, more red blood cells, higher rate of basal metabolism and respiratory rate and a greater concentration of haemoglobin in the blood.

Hormones also work on secondary sexual characteristics, influencing voice change and beard and body hair growth in boys. In girls, sex hormones are responsible for breast development and the regular pattern of sex hormones that govern the menstrual cycle. There is no equivalent cycle in boys. The differences established at adolescence between boys and girls follow into adulthood.

Proportionality

Alterations in body proportions accompany changes in height and weight, and growth is not simply an increase in size but influences the contribution different body parts make to overall shape.

As a general rule, the body grows in an orderly and predictable fashion but the speed at which these changes occur is different for everyone. In all children, there are three general directions of growth.

1   Early in life, growth is fastest in the head area and slower in body parts further away from the head. The relatively large head of the newborn and young child compared with arms and legs illustrates this. Infants develop muscular control over the head and neck before they can voluntarily use lower parts of the body.

2   Growth also occurs more in the trunk, and then progressively in the arms and legs. Children can control the larger muscles of the body, arms and thighs before they can master sophisticated movements using their fingers and toes.

3   The back part of the body grows and develops faster than the front. For example, the spinal area is well developed at birth and provides a sound base for normal neuromuscular development.

51

Even though changes to the proportions of the body are governed by different periods of slow or more rapid growth and the timing of maturity differs between individuals, overall growth is steady and continuous.

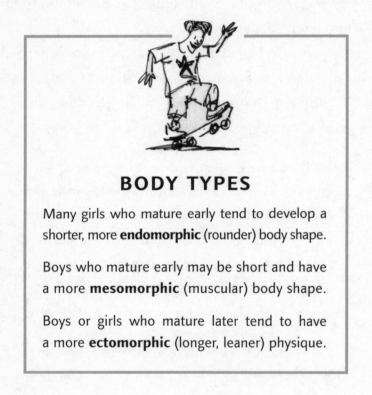

BODY TYPES

Many girls who mature early tend to develop a shorter, more **endomorphic** (rounder) body shape.

Boys who mature early may be short and have a more **mesomorphic** (muscular) body shape.

Boys or girls who mature later tend to have a more **ectomorphic** (longer, leaner) physique.

Key features of growth and development

Infancy

Defined as immediately after birth and for the first year (some definitions also include the second year), infancy is the most explosive period of growth, with dramatic increases in height, weight and the development of the nervous system. Coordination and mental processes also develop rapidly during infancy.

During the initial days of life, while they are only taking in small quantities of highly concentrated colostrum, a newborn baby loses some weight due to urine losses. This is normal. Once the mother's breast milk 'comes in' on about the third day, the baby gradually gains weight. The baby usually regains its birth-weight by about the end of the first week. A steady gain in weight then occurs, although the rate of gain varies with the individual baby.

During the first three months, the average baby gains about 1 kg a month. By 6 months of age, the average gain has dropped to 0.5 kg per month. By the end of the first year, most babies have tripled their birth weight, but then they slow down, gaining only about 2.5 kg during the second year. Babies also grow 25–30 cm in length (height) in their first year and a further 12 cm in the second year. Babies continue to deposit extra body fat, usually peaking at about 9 months.

Childhood

It ends when puberty begins, with the timing varying in different children. Growth during childhood is steady but generally relatively slow compared with infancy, except for periods of peak height velocity during which a child may grow more in a year than at any time other than during infancy. Each year, the average child grows approximately 5–6 cm and increases weight by 2.3 kg.

Adolescence

Adolescence begins at puberty when secondary sexual characteristics appear and the reproductive system matures. Body composition also changes and many psychological and

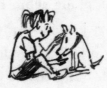

Physical changes

GIRLS	10–11	•breast buds form •start of growth spurt •sparse pubic hair
	11–14	•more pubic hair •rapid growth of reproductive organs, including ovaries, uterus and vagina •menarche •breasts enlarge •age of maximum growth
	14–16	•underarm hair grows to complement pubic growth •breasts grow to adult size and shape
BOYS	11.5–13	•initial growth of testes and scrotum •sparse pubic hair •start of growth spurt •growth of penis
	13–16	•continued growth of pubic hair •voice becomes deeper •maturation of reproductive organs including the penis, testes, scrotum and associated glands •initial facial hair •age of maximum growth
	16–18	•growth in bodily hair •voice becomes deeper

emotional adjustments occur. Rapid changes occur, but at different ages, depending on the individual. There is no 'normal' age for adolescence, although the physical growth changes of puberty are orderly and predictable in each individual.

During childhood, boys and girls have many physical similarities. During late childhood, girls grow rapidly in height — their time of peak height growth rate. This occurs about 18 months to 2 years earlier in the average girl compared with boys and gives girls a slight size advantage at this time. The appearance of breast buds and then peak height velocity are the first physical signs of puberty in girls and a rapid increase in height is the best sign that a girl is approaching menarche when her first menstruation will occur.

The average girl experiences peak growth rate for height at 11.8 years of age and the most common time to reach menarche is 12.8 years. However, individual girls differ and a range of 2 years is common.

Growth of the testes is the best early sign of puberty in boys. Their peak growth rate occurs at about 14 years of age and is longer than that of girls. The average adult man is 12–13 cm taller than the average woman and about 8–10 cm of this height difference is because boys have a longer growth period that allows for longer limbs. The other 3–5 cm height difference is due to boys' higher peak growth rate compared with girls.

The speed with which children grow and reach their final adult size varies. Some children are more physically mature at the same chronological age. However, even though a child who is an early developer will reach adult status earlier, the final height of a late developer may be similar to the early maturer. Some overweight children are tall for their age, have a more advanced skeletal age, reach puberty earlier and may have a high lean body mass. Growth usually stops between age 16 and the early 20s, although some bones do not stop growing until well into early adulthood. Some girls may appear to finish growing earlier, but growth changes in bones may continue even without any obvious increase in height.

The influence of genes

Growth and body type or physique is influenced by inherited and environmental factors. Genes provide a blueprint for the potential for growth and environmental factors, including health, nutrition and physical activity, and determine the degree to which the inherited potential is reached.

Although genes can't be altered, physical shape can be changed by environmental conditions such as stringent dietary restriction, over-consumption combined with inactivity, or an increase in muscle mass from a weight-training program.

Body composition

Body fat

Body weight is mainly made up of water, fat, bone and muscle. All these components of the body are normal and desirable. Water is essential for all body functions. After age 4, boys have a greater percentage of their body weight as water — largely because they carry less body fat.

Fat protects vital organs and governs external shape and appearance. Much of our body fat exists as deposits under the surface of the skin (subcutaneous fat). Very low levels of body fat are undesirable and can compromise the essential levels of fat needed for normal bodily functions. Low body fat levels can interfere with normal menstrual function in girls and very low levels of body fat can also interfere with the growth of bones and muscle. As a guide, the minimum safe levels of body fat for teenagers would be 12% for girls and 6% for boys.

Skinfold thickness indicates how much subcutaneous fat is present. As with all aspects of physical growth, changes in skinfold thickness vary in individual children. However, subcutaneous fat indicates overall fatness. The average teenage girl has significantly more subcutaneous fat than the average boy, particularly around the pelvis, breasts, upper back and arms, giving a more rounded appearance. Between 14–16 years of age, girls average 21–23% body fat. Boys average 10–12% fat. These values are used as indicators of appropriate body fat levels at this age.

Female fashion models are usually very tall and have slender hips and buttocks. Some people assume this is normal, but the shape of models is desirable because it is unusual. Fat on the hips and buttocks is much less of a health hazard than fat around the waist, which is associated with an increased risk of type 2 diabetes and other health problems in adults.

The differences in subcutaneous fat have other effects on physical appearance. Men are more muscular than women, and the lower subcutaneous fat levels make men's muscles more prominent. This is one reason why athletic girls with well-developed skeletal muscles do not look as muscular as boys.

Fat cells

There are times in life when the number of fat cells in the body can increase rapidly. These include the period before birth and during infancy and adolescence. Between birth and about 6 years of age, both boys and girls have an increase in their number of fat cells (known as hyperplasia). After about age 8, fat deposits tend to fill out the existing fat cells although children who become obese also continue to produce new fat cells. Such increases in fat cell numbers may also occur in obese adults. The potential for a continuing increase in the number of fat cells helps explain why some people who become obese find it difficult to lose weight.

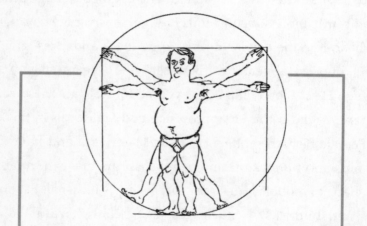

HYPERTROPHY

Fat cells can fill up with fat at any age and stage of life and this is the main way body fat levels increase after puberty. An increase in the size of fat cells is known as hypertrophy.

There does not seem to be any way of decreasing the number of existing fat cells in the body, other than with surgery, so those who already have an increased number of fat cells will carry them for the rest of their lives. However, it is possible to reduce the amount of fat in each fat cell by losing weight.

Muscle

The size and shape of the developing body, including the relationship between fat and muscle, can have important repercussions for children and teenagers. A child who is more muscular has advantages in physical activity that may carry over to the social setting. On the other hand, children who carry more weight may be at a disadvantage. This can become worse if their extra weight causes difficulty with some movement and poor development of motor skills, which then means they have less opportunity to participate in activities compared with children of normal weight.

Growth of muscles increases throughout the growing years and reaches a peak about three months after reaching peak height velocity. Increases in strength lag behind growth changes by a similar period. Differences in strength during the pre-pubertal years are generally not great, but boys tend to be stronger, possibly because they are exposed to more physical activities that encourage strength. For a short period, some girls who reach puberty earlier may be stronger than some boys.

3

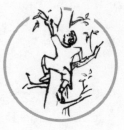

Measuring up

Many people judge overweight or obesity by looking at the child. This can be useful, especially for an experienced doctor or dietitian, but the modern desire for extreme slimness means that many normal-sized children now judge themselves to be overweight. A more objective assessment is preferable.

Information about the percentage of body fat can be a useful guide during a child's growing years, providing measurements are accurate and you can compare results with what is normal. However, after infancy, such details can also lead to an undesirable preoccupation with body fat.

Normal levels of body fat vary with age. At birth, approximately 12% of body weight is present as fat. This rises rapidly and peaks at about 6 months of age when 25% of an infant's body is fat. Levels then fall over the next 10 years to about 17–18% body fat content, changing again at puberty when boys lose fat and girls gain some.

Differences between the sexes are influenced by various factors, including nutrition and individual variation, so generalised comparisons are really only valid for large numbers of people at similar levels of fatness. As mentioned in Chapter 2, minimum safe levels in teenagers are 12% for girls and 6% for boys; average levels are 21–23% for girls and 10–12% for boys 14–16 years of age. Levels of body fat above 25% for boys and 32% for girls are considered excessive.

Charts for parents

Height/weight charts are only suitable as a rough guide to weight status. Use them with caution, especially if they appear

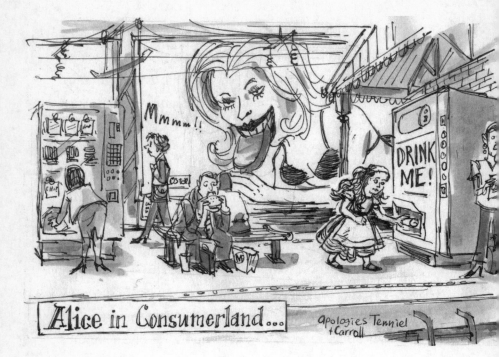

Alice in Consumerland...

in a magazine or on an Internet site that has not been endorsed by a recognised expert. Check what data have been used to compile the chart and that they apply to a relevant societal group. For example, using data from Europe or the United States would not be relevant in some Asian countries.

Some charts ask you to nominate a frame size, usually offering 'small', 'medium' or 'large' as choices. However, there is no easy way for the average person to determine frame size. Some people also 'adjust' frame size — for example, those with a medium frame size who do not fit the desirable weight range for that frame may classify themselves as having a 'large frame'. Frame sizes do vary, but many people who think they have a large frame are amazed how much smaller their frame appears to be once they have lost excess body fat.

Growth charts published by groups such as the National Health and Medical Research Council (see pages 65 and 66) are better indicators of height and weight, but need to be related to a child's age and stage of development.

Charts for professionals

If children's height, weight and skinfold thickness measurements are recorded at different times, they can provide a useful record of physical changes. The percentage of body weight made up of fat can be measured or calculated from measurements of skinfold thickness at a number of sites around the body. However, this method relies on accurate measurements so should only be used by those who are well trained. Textbooks also give details of more complicated laboratory methods that can be used to assess body composition, although most are not available to the general public.

The Body Mass Index

Strictly speaking, the BMI doesn't measure fatness. However, it is useful as a guide to health status. It extends the idea of height–weight charts using a formula that has been found to correspond well with the risk of common health problems — at least on a population basis. For children, it needs to be compared with age-related values representative of normal healthy children who are considered to be of normal size. The BMI is calculated by dividing weight (in kilograms) by height squared (in metres).

63

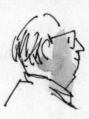

SEE A PROFESSIONAL

Medical doctors or health professionals qualified in nutrition and weight control can objectively and accurately assess whether a child is overweight or obese. They can also give family members an insight into strategies to change various aspects of lifestyle. The whole family can benefit from learning about the advantages of regular physical activity and good eating habits.

How to work it out

Let's take a couple of examples:

- A person who weighs 45 kg and is 1.5 m tall. Their height, 1.5, squared (1.5 x 1.5) is 2.25.

- Their weight, 45, divided by 2.25, gives a BMI of 20.

- Someone who weighs 67.5 kg, but is the same height, would have a BMI of 30: 67.5 ÷ 2.25 = 30.

For those over 18 years of age, a BMI between 25 and 29.9 is defined as overweight, while a BMI greater than 30 is defined as obese. Data for children also include a factor related to their age.

2 to 20 years: Boys
Body mass index-for-age percentiles

NAME _____

RECORD # _____

Date	Age	Weight	Stature	BMI*	Comments

*To Calculate BMI: Weight (kg) ÷ Stature (cm) ÷ Stature (cm) x 10,000
or Weight (lb) ÷ Stature (in) ÷ Stature (in) x 703

BMI

35
34
33
32
31
30
29
28
27
26
25
24
23
22
21
20
19
18
17
16
15
14
13
12

BMI
27
26
25
24
23
22
21
20
19
18
17
16
15
14
13
12

95
90
85
75
50
25
10
5

kg/m²

AGE (YEARS)

kg/m²

2   3   4   5   6   7   8   9   10   11   12   13   14   15   16   17   18   19   20

Published May 30, 2000 (modified 10/16/00).

SOURCE: Developed by the National Center for Health Statistics in collaboration with
the National Center for Chronic Disease Prevention and Health Promotion (2000).
http://www.cdc.gov/growthcharts

CDC

SAFER · HEALTHIER · PEOPLE™

65

2 to 20 years: Girls
Body mass index-for-age percentiles

NAME _____

RECORD # _____

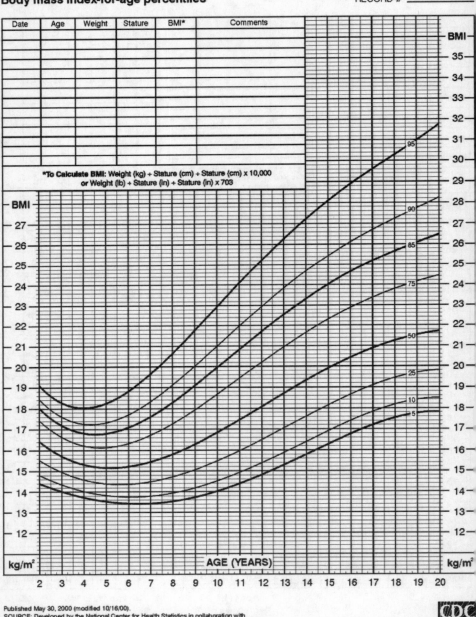

*To Calculate BMI: Weight (kg) ÷ Stature (cm) ÷ Stature (cm) x 10,000
or Weight (lb) ÷ Stature (in) ÷ Stature (in) x 703

Published May 30, 2000 (modified 10/16/00).
SOURCE: Developed by the National Center for Health Statistics in collaboration with
the National Center for Chronic Disease Prevention and Health Promotion (2000).
http://www.cdc.gov/growthcharts

4

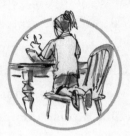

Changing
perceptions

Body image

What is considered desirable (in terms of body size) varies between individuals and is influenced by culture, ethnicity, family background, sex, socio-economic status and fashion. In old movies, actors, models and screen goddesses were fatter than what is considered desirable now. Looking at famous paintings, we can see that many artists also preferred to paint voluptuous women and well-rounded children. This may have been related to the prevailing ideals of beauty or to the fact that those who were well-rounded had access to sufficient food and were more likely to be from the upper classes. By contrast, the preferred body shape of men seems not to have changed over the centuries. Our society currently worships slenderness in women and approves of men with well-formed muscles and little body fat.

Slim images abound, promoted by the media, advertising agencies and fashion designers. The media play a powerful role in the current preoccupation with body weight and extreme slimness, and some seem to ignore the risk to the health of children and teenagers who are confronted with images of supposed perfection that are unattainable by the average person. These images have always been presented more to girls than boys, although men's magazines and advertisements are beginning to encourage boys to think there is something wrong with their bodies if they are not represented by the 'six-pack' musculature considered desirable by advertisers.

Society's attitudes define obesity. This is a major reason why children — whatever their weight — devalue an obese body and also why so many girls and an increasing number of boys feel dissatisfied with their bodies. Both boys and girls think girls must be thin to be acceptable, while many boys are now being encouraged to feel dissatisfaction with their own bodies unless they are tall and muscular. These unrealistic ideals are leading many people to spend a lifetime fighting against their body form and shape, including those aspects that are genetically determined and over which they have no control.

Our perception of our physical selves — our body image — influences the way we feel, and vice versa. When things are going well and a child or teenager with a poor body image is in good spirits, he or she may be relatively untroubled by the disability, although the problem may not be far below the surface. When things are not going so well, unpleasant experiences can surface and reduce self-esteem further, reinforcing a disturbed body image. The intensity of disturbances in body image can fluctuate widely, even over short periods of time. (In adults, disturbances of body image tend to persist with remarkably little change over time. This is why not all obese adults who lose weight enjoy significant psychological improvement. Their disturbance of body image is too ingrained, often to their surprise and dismay.)

Some experts report that most body image disturbances occur in those who became obese during childhood and adolescence. These people have a preoccupation with their condition, as occurs in anorexia nervosa. However, it is a mistake to assume all obese people are psychologically or emotionally disturbed.

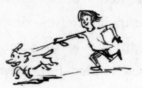

SETTING A GOOD EXAMPLE

Adults who fear fatness and are preoccupied with body weight and body fat encourage children and teenagers to think the same way. When a child's mother is constantly dieting or overly concerned about her own weight, her daughters have a higher than usual rate of dieting and developing eating disorders. Rather than dwelling on weight itself, it would help if parents set a good example by eating and drinking healthily and ensuring they enjoyed plenty of physical activity.

AN ELUSIVE GOAL

Thinness is often associated with being healthy and encourages many people, both fat and thin, to pursue or maintain a thin body image. While it's true that many thin people are healthy, those who achieve thinness by semi-starvation or by following diets that do not provide enough nutrients are often unhealthy.

Our society exalts tall, lean and more athletic looking people and often ridicules those who are obese, even making some feel like social outcasts. Children and teenagers are especially cruel in this way and can put pressure on each other while they are very young. Because of this societal attitude, many children and teenagers carry a substantial social and psychological burden that their bodies are not 'perfect' enough. Many high-school students, particularly girls, think they are overweight even when all objective measures show they are not. Such distortions of body image and the psychological problems associated with them are a major factor that can lead a small percentage of teenagers to develop eating disorders.

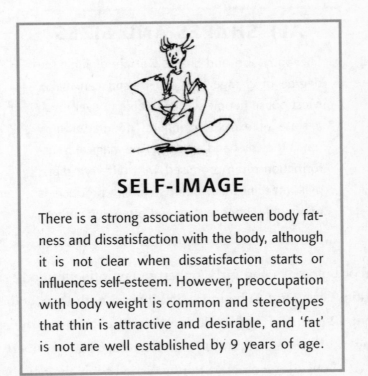

SELF-IMAGE

There is a strong association between body fatness and dissatisfaction with the body, although it is not clear when dissatisfaction starts or influences self-esteem. However, preoccupation with body weight is common and stereotypes that thin is attractive and desirable, and 'fat' is not are well established by 9 years of age.

Differences between boys and girls

Overweight and obese girls may have less confidence in their physical appearance and athletic competence than their normal-weight peers, but body weight doesn't necessarily impact on how girls rate their self-esteem. Heavier girls are less likely to be nominated by their peers as pretty, although this does not necessarily affect their popularity.

Boys are generally more satisfied than girls with their physical appearance, although teenage boys and girls are less satisfied if they perceive themselves as 'fat'. Boys generally wish they were more muscular, while girls want to be thinner. More boys think they are too thin and more girls believe they are too fat.

ALL SHAPES AND SIZES

The body size and shape we inherit limit the degree of change that any person can make. Most obese people will be unable to ever reach a state of extreme thinness, no matter how much they diet and exercise. The magical transformation often promised with different diets, pills, machines and other slimming products is impossible, unnecessary and often unhealthy.

For both boys and girls, puberty may influence body satisfaction. Girls tend to be more dissatisfied with their bodies at about 12 years of age while boys don't experience the same thing until they are about 14 — their average age of puberty. By age 16, boys are generally more satisfied with their bodies as they move towards their mature adult physique, while girls continue to be dissatisfied with their appearance. The numbers of overweight boys and girls are fairly equal but nearly twice as many girls see themselves as overweight compared with boys.

More girls than boys say they exercise for weight control and to improve their body tone. Those who exercise for fitness, health and enjoyment report less disturbance in their body image, but those who exercise for weight control, tone and attractiveness have greater dissatisfaction with their bodies.

Pressures on teenagers

Body image describes our attitude and feeling towards our bodies. It is a dynamic concept and is constantly affected by new experiences and activities. Height, weight, body build, facial characteristics and other features that normally change throughout life are all associated with body image.

In young children, changes in appearance and overall body size are usually easily absorbed into the total body image. But during puberty and throughout adolescence, the dramatic and rapid changes in size, body proportions, body composition, and primary and secondary sexual characteristics can't be accommodated by minor adjustments in body image. This leads most teenagers to experience a conscious and major change in their body image.

With the increasing prevalence of overweight and obesity, body fatness and weight loss are important issues in the community, but some teenagers whose weight is normal or even below the healthy weight range want to be thinner. This can lead to a preoccupation with dieting.

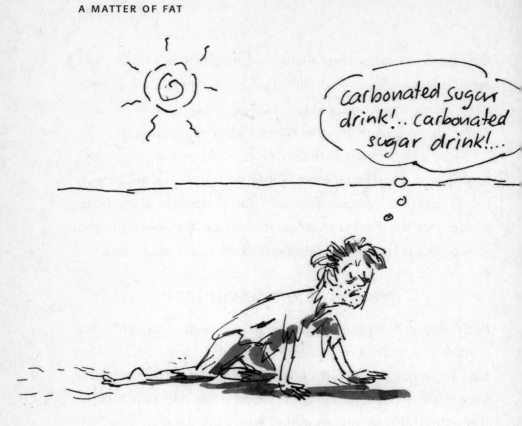

Dieting and fasting

Diets

Many people think dieting is an easy answer to obesity. In fact, most diets are unsuitable for children and are rarely successful long-term at any age. Trying to eat as little as possible or following some unbalanced diet deprives children and teenagers of the high nutrient levels needed for growth and normal development. Going on a diet can lead to a preoccupation with body weight that is psychologically unhealthy. Diets are perceived as negative and other children (and adults) may make derogatory remarks about people on diets that can make the overweight child feel as though he or she is different. For long-term control of body fat levels, diets should usually be avoided and substituted with healthier happy eating and exercise habits for the whole family. The only way to lose weight and keep it off permanently is to change the eating and exercise habits that caused the problem in the first place.

Many unsuccessful attempts to lose weight and keep it off can make each further attempt to lose weight more difficult. This is a major reason why parents should take preventive action at a young age when it is easier to encourage good eating and exercise habits in growing children. Changing entrenched habits is much more difficult, although it can be done.

The latest diet can bring great profits for magazines and the authors of diet books. These diets vary dramatically. Depending on the fad of the moment, they may be high or low in fat, protein or carbohydrate. There are many foolish and unbalanced diets and a lot of rubbish is written about weight-loss. Some impose strict rules about what you can eat and drink. Others are designed to sell supplements, powders, drinks or some snack that is intended to replace meals. Most claim to be *the* way to lose weight quickly and easily. New diets appear with monotonous regularity and many make dieting sound easy and promise fast results.

In general, it's fair to say that any change in food consumption that reduces kilojoules will result in weight-loss — at least while you stick to the diet. Most diets don't work in the long term because almost no one can keep eating the restricted range of foods most of them permit. Once most people go off a diet, they regain most of what they lost. It is much more important to learn appropriate eating and exercise habits that will last a lifetime.

Some sellers of diets, supplements or drugs to treat obesity claim many varied reasons why people gain excess body fat. Their theories are unproven and there is no escaping the fact that excess body fat only accumulates if more kilojoules of energy come into the body from food and drink than are used for growth, metabolism and physical activity. The body can store excess kilojoules as deposits of fat. Dietary fats can be easily converted to body fat. Carbohydrates are less easily converted to fat and are preferentially used by the body for energy. However, if carbohydrate intake is excessive, any fats that are consumed will not be used for energy and will end up as body fat deposits.

Reject any diet that makes the following claims:

- fast weight-loss;

- no effort is required;

- new or revolutionary;

- no exercise is needed;

- has a magic ingredient;

- special powders, pills or meal replacement products are necessary;

- you can eat whatever you like with this product;

- whole food groups such as breads, cereals and grains, or all fats or carbohydrates are unnecessary;

- you can eat unlimited amounts of fats or meats, cheeses or any other food;

- special wraps, garments, passive exercise machines (where you do nothing), injections or supplements will help weight-loss;

- only one particular range of foods, with no substitutions allowed, will be effective;

- you can eat lots of kilojoules and still lose weight.

Many popular diets are especially unsuitable for growing children because they do not provide the nutrients needed for children's growth and to protect their future health. Before using any diet for children, ask your doctor or a dietitian or other health professional who has no vested interest in the diet being promoted whether it is appropriate. Chapter 5 has details of healthy eating habits for children.

Losing weight takes time

Too often people have unreal expectations of the way the body can change its weight or shape. Diets and some fitness programs make this worse by promising quick and easy results. Change takes time, however. Excess weight accumulates because of an energy imbalance over an extended period and it takes time to change this. Drastic attempts to lose weight are fraught with all sorts of pitfalls. Even when your doctor says weight loss is a medical goal, the weight loss should be gradual. Fast weight loss is almost always followed by fast regaining of the weight lost. When this occurs, most people think there is some problem within themselves that has caused the failure. In fact, it is usually the diet that was at fault.

Don't use the scales too often

It's tempting for people who are trying to do something about their weight to weigh themselves often. This is not wise. Body weight normally fluctuates during the day, depending mainly on fluid balance, but also on when you have eaten or been to the toilet. It is therefore best to monitor body weight not more than once a week — and preferably less often — rather than taking much notice of daily fluctuations.

When people weigh themselves too often, they feel elated if the scales record a lower reading and may become depressed if there is no change or an increase. Body fat is burnt slowly and these fluctuations are therefore meaningless, at best. At worst, someone who appears to be losing lots of weight may give themselves more 'treats' and someone who does not appear to be successful may take comfort in food. It is better not to place so much reliance on the scales, especially for children who may develop a hatred of what the scales say. For some overweight children, it may be best not to weigh them at home, although it is useful for the local doctor to keep records of the child's weight over the years.

A time of change

The transition from childhood to adolescence is a time of great change, with girls' bodies increasing in fat as they change from that of a child to that of a mature young woman. Some young women involved in sport face a dilemma with biological changes in their size and shape co-existing with a desire to control their eating and weight for appearance and performance.

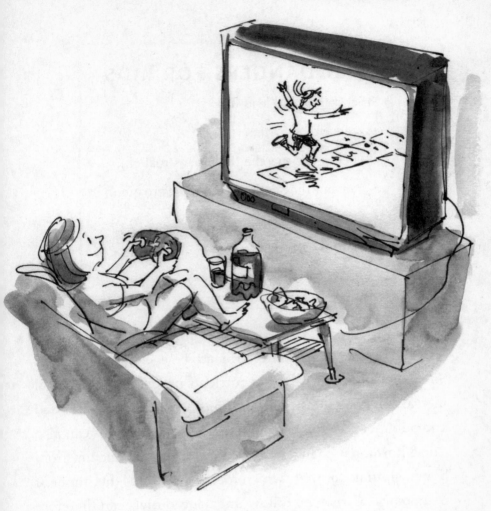

Some girls who diet are overweight, but many are of normal weight or even underweight. Some are so preoccupied with body size, shape, weight and fatness that they diet or exercise inappropriately, sometimes abusing their bodies in the process. Preoccupation with losing weight can play a role in eating and weight disorders, including obesity. Some diets are so stringent that few people can stand them for long, 'breaking out' to binge eat as a result of the deprivation of the diet. Many teenagers, especially girls, alternate strict dieting with overeating.

DIET DANGERS FOR KIDS

Strict dieting can lead to:

- retarded growth;

- delayed menarche (first menstruation);

- amenorrhoea (absence of menstruation);

- loss of muscle;

- future osteoporosis;

- psychological disturbances.

Dieting can cause long-term adverse effects on bones. Some diets don't provide the nutrients needed for the normal increase in bone density that should occur during childhood and adolescence. To make matters worse, strict diets can also cause hormonal changes that lead to a loss of calcium from bone, similar to that which occurs around the time of menopause. Girls who follow unbalanced diets can therefore put themselves at high risk of future osteoporosis by not developing strong bones and also starting loss of calcium many years earlier than occurs when women have to cope with calcium loss after age 50.

Most behaviours are part of a continuum and dieting is no exception. At one extreme, there are those who don't diet and at the other are those with an eating disorder. In between, there are varying levels of dieting. Not all who diet develop eating disorders, but since dieting is a common prelude to anorexia and bulimia nervosa, binge eating and weight cycling, it should therefore be seen as problematic behaviour. Dieting during childhood and adolescence is a special worry as the highest incidence of anorexia nervosa occurs at the beginning of adolescence. Bulimia nervosa is more common at the end of adolescence.

Fasting

Fasting is not a good way for anyone to try to lose weight and is especially undesirable for children and teenagers. The body does not distinguish the different intent between fasting and starvation and when a person doesn't eat, the body cuts back the energy it uses for metabolism and physical activity and goes into low energy survival mode. Fasting can adversely affect growth and deprives the body of essential nutrients. There is no evidence that fasting is useful for long-term weight-loss and the cut-back in metabolic rate with fasting means it can be counter-productive for those trying to lose weight. After a fast, most people also overeat.

Eating disorders

The term 'eating disorder' usually refers to **anorexia nervosa**, **bulimia nervosa** or **binge eating**. Strictly speaking, obesity can also be defined as an eating or weight disorder. Eating and weight disorders are complex, but seem to be more common in those who lack self-esteem and a sense of effectiveness. They are also often associated with an unrealistically thin body image.

The exact causes of eating disorders are not known, but risk factors include:

- family influences;
- genetic predisposition;
- biological mechanisms;
- personality and individual psychopathology.

Psychological events related to the onset of anorexia nervosa can include:

- extreme disappointment about the failure of or problems with an important relationship;
- the birth of a sibling;
- moving house;
- the loss of a friend;
- a death in the family.

Physical events may include:

- early physical maturation;
- anxiety about puberty.

Those with an eating disorder are often secretive and manipulative in their behaviour. Bulimia nervosa may cause victims to be secretive, feel guilty, have low self-esteem and be angry about their incapacity to control how much they eat.

Less than 1% of the population have anorexia nervosa, with bulimia affecting 1–3%. Many more people have eating and weight-related problems, including dieting and binge-eating, but do not meet strict diagnostic criteria for an eating disorder. About a quarter of those who seek treatment for obesity have periodic bouts of binge eating. Obese binge-eaters may have failed often in their attempts to lose weight and follow each dieting period by abandoning all dietary restraint. These people tend to be more dissatisfied with their weight and are more preoccupied with their weight and food than other obese people.

Common problems include:

- an unhealthy preoccupation with weight and food;

- crash diets;

- obsessive thinking about weight;

- disturbed body image.

Can concern about obesity lead to eating disorders? Statistics about the incidence of eating and weight disorders in different populations are confusing, partly due to different definitions. Because anorexia nervosa often attracts media coverage, some assume it is more common than is the case and want to downplay concern about excess weight in case it induces anorexia nervosa. All extremes of body weight may lead to impaired health and should be avoided, but it is important to keep the incidence of each in perspective. Currently about a quarter of teenage girls are overweight — many times the number suffering from an eating disorder. There is no evidence that community concern about obesity and promotion of a healthy weight — which is neither too high nor too low — leads to eating disorders.

When over-nutrition is combined with low levels of physical activity, or under-nutrition is combined with excessive physical activity, the risk of an eating or weight disorder increases. In sports such as gymnastics, dancing, diving, skating, swimming and endurance events, where leanness is highly prized and important for success, athletes are at high risk of an eating disorder.

Anorexia and bulimia nervosa are complex, closely-related alterations in eating behaviour, both related to an underlying fear of 'fatness'.

Anorexia nervosa

In anorexia, there is weight loss, poor body image and an intense fear of weight gain, especially what is seen as the 'fatness' of the normal mature female body that starts at puberty. Excessive physical activity is also a common symptom.

Official diagnostic criteria

1 Refusal to maintain body weight at or above a minimally normal weight for age and height. For example, weight loss or failure to gain weight according to growth, so that body weight is less than 85% of expected weight.

2 Intense fears of gaining weight or becoming fat even though underweight.

3 Disturbance in the perception of body weight or shape with an undue influence on self-evaluation, or denial of the seriousness of low body weight.

4 If periods have started, the absence of at least three consecutive menstrual cycles.

Bulimia

Bulimia may occur in conjunction with anorexia or on its own, and may be associated with normal weight, underweight or overweight. Like anorexia, it is also characterised by an intense fear of fatness. Those with bulimia may binge on large quantities of food at one time and then purge this by vomiting or taking laxatives or diuretics, or they may fast or engage in excessive exercise. Bulimia may also be stimulated by strict diets.

Purging and vomiting are hazardous features of bulimia nervosa and may also occur in anorexia nervosa. Both deprive the body of needed nutrients and have adverse psychological effects. There is a higher incidence of purging behaviour in children who have been sexually abused and anyone of any age who deliberately and repeatedly vomits needs professional help. Dentists often pick up cases of bulimia nervosa because the acidity of vomit damages tooth enamel. Bulimia nervosa can also damage the oesophagus.

Official diagnostic criteria

1 Recurrent episodes of binge eating, characterised by:

(a) eating an amount of food that is much larger than most people would eat during a similar period of time (say a 2-hour period) and under similar circumstances;

(b) a feeling of lack of control over eating where you feel you can't stop or control what or how much you are eating.

2 Recurrent inappropriate compensatory behaviour to prevent weight gain, such as self-induced vomiting, misuse of laxatives, diuretics, enemas or other medications, fasting, excessive exercise.

3 Binge eating and inappropriate compensatory behaviours occurring on average at least twice a week for 3 months.

4 Self-evaluation being unduly influenced by body shape and weight.

5 The disturbance does not occur just during episodes of anorexia nervosa.

Binge-eating disorder (BED)

Binges may be precipitated by negative emotions and feeling out-of-control. When binge eaters feel guilty, they may follow the binge with increased dietary restraint that perpetuates an unbalanced relationship with food.

Official diagnostic criteria

1 Recurrent episodes of binge eating. An episode of binge eating is characterised by:
(a) eating an amount of food that is much larger than most people would eat in a similar period of time (say a 2-hour period) and under similar circumstances;
(b) a feeling of lack of control while eating where you feel you can't stop or control what or how much you are eating.

2   The binge-eating episodes are associated with three (or more) of the following:

(a) eating much more rapidly than normal;

(b) eating until you feel uncomfortably full;

(c) eating large amounts of food when you are not feeling physically hungry;

(d) eating alone because of being embarrassed by how much you are eating;

(e) feeling disgusted with yourself, depressed, or very guilty after overeating.

3   Marked distress about binge eating.

4   The binge eating occurs, on average, at least 2 days a week for 6 months.

5   The binge eating is not associated with the regular use of inappropriate compensatory behaviours such as purging, fasting or excessive exercise, and does not occur exclusively during the course of anorexia nervosa or bulimia nervosa.

Understanding and support

Anyone who has an eating and weight disorder or eating-disordered behaviour needs help. Knowing and understanding the person concerned and planning a support program is vital for prevention, treatment and management. For anyone with anorexia nervosa, the goals should include gaining some weight. For those with bulimia, or obese people with binge-eating disorder, keeping weight stable may be more important. Treatment should always be tailored to the unique developmental, medical, nutritional and psychological needs of the person concerned.

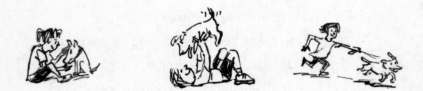

Building confidence

Exercise

From an early age, we need to promote exercise as a way to achieve health and wellness, rather than using exercise just as a way to control weight. Exercise may be useful and adolescents with anorexia may benefit from individualised resistance training sessions to preserve and strengthen skeletal muscle tissue.

Once they reach school age, children who are obese may be vulnerable and sensitive to the comments of their peers. For some, the associated social stigma turns them off participating in sport and social activities, with many dreading involvement in any activities where people are watching.

Involvement in non-threatening physical activities can overcome such fears and families can help by introducing enjoyable activities that lead to an increase in regular physical activity. When children participate and are successful in any physical activity, they are more likely to continue with it.

Activity classes specifically for obese children sometimes provide an environment that may be more conducive to participation, although some children may feel stigmatised by joining such a group.

Everyone likes being successful and obese children are no different. Once children improve their motor fitness, they are more likely to gain enough self-confidence to return to regular physical education and sport without it being a traumatic experience.

Overcoming stereotypes

One common belief is that overweight people are lazy, gluttonous and lack will power and self-control. In fact, there is no proof that overweight children fit any of these stereotypes. However, the psychological and social problems associated with obesity can be as serious as the medical hazards. Those who are obese have to cope with the social stigma attached to their appearance and many will then take solace from food and eat for compensation and comfort. In some cases, especially in teenagers, the reverse may occur and food can become an object of hatred and disdain, possibly leading to eating disorders such as anorexia nervosa or bulimia nervosa. To counteract such problems, try to encourage children's self-esteem and build their confidence in themselves as worthwhile people.

Encouraging high self-esteem, self-confidence and sound body image is essential throughout childhood. The longer problems related to body weight go unchecked, the greater the risk of future problems. Unfortunately, the self-esteem and self-confidence obese children need may be lacking because of their past experiences. Those who see themselves as ugly or unattractive to others may be unhappy and depressed. It is vitally important to help obese children avoid experiencing the life-long misery and dissatisfaction that occurs in those who hate their bodies and become preoccupied with their weight.

To help children with self-esteem:

- value and listen attentively to their thoughts and viewpoints;

- accept their ideas and contributions as valid;

- be honest with them;

- foster an understanding that everyone is different. We don't all end up the same height or have the same size feet and neither will we all be the same weight or shape. Show an appreciation that many sizes and shapes make up a definition of normal;

- discourage dieting and constant weighing (get rid of bathroom scales);

- encourage a 'can do' approach to healthy eating and exercise for the whole family.

It may also be important to seek professional advice and support from a psychologist or dietitian who has experience working with young people. Parents may sometimes be too close to the problem and may use wrong tactics, involving a 'shame and blame' thought process.

Support groups are valuable for some children and for their families. In general, if one family member has a problem, the whole family needs to make appropriate changes.

Emotional factors

It is easy to use food as a comfort. Some children who are worried about an aspect of their schooling or their relationship with friends or peers may take comfort in eating. Learn ways to comfort and reward children other than with food. For example, take small children for a walk to a park or make time to play with them or read a book rather than offering them a biscuit or chocolate. Older children may appreciate you helping them with some chore, arranging a canoe trip or a horse ride or going and helping someone else in the community.

Education

Both parents and teachers need to be vigilant in stressing a sensible approach to nutrition and physical activity and teach young people the facts about physical growth and the inevitability of individual differences in body size and shape.

For children or adolescents who are genuinely too fat, any advice about fat loss should come under the supervision of a qualified dietitian. Chapter 5 gives details of safe and healthy eating for those who need to lose body fat.

5

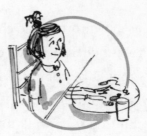

Food

Food was once relatively simple. Our human ancestors ate what was available and were happy if the quantity available was sufficient. Until recently, food remained relatively simple and children ate what their parents ate, suitably chopped, mashed or even chewed, until they had teeth. Until supermarkets took off in the 1960s, we had about 600 foods to choose from, many available only in season. The modern supermarket now stocks 12–15,000 foods, including 1,750 different snack foods!

No one can sample everything in the modern supermarket so we now make food choices according to many factors. Rather than giving kids what we eat, we now have special foods for them and children themselves exert great influence over their own and the family's food choices.

When children begin eating solid foods, factors influencing food choice include:

- whether they are breast-fed;
- the foods available;
- age, activity and growth rate;
- the foods they are accustomed to;
- whether they eat regular family foods or are given special foods;
- individual taste preferences;
- parents' time constraints;
- where they eat (with the family, on their own, at childcare or in the car);
- advice from family and friends;

- peer group pressure;

- advertising (directed at mothers or children);

- television (programs as well as advertising).

Healthy eating habits at different ages and stages

Infants

The first influence on children's dietary behaviour comes from warm, sweet breast milk that changes in flavour every feed, depending on what the mother has been eating. Breast-fed babies drink varying amounts, according to their physiological needs. Since the mother does not really know how much the baby has consumed, breast-fed babies adjust their appetite according to what they need at the time rather than consuming a set amount at each feed. There is evidence that breast-fed babies are less likely to become obese or develop allergies.

STRATEGIES FOR PARENTS

Breast-feed, if possible. The World Health Organisation's guidelines recommend breast milk as a child's sole food for the first 6 months of life.

- For babies who are not breast-fed, an appropriate infant formula should be given while the baby is held closely.

- The mother or carer should respect variations in the baby's appetite rather than encouraging the baby to consume a set quantity at each feed.

- Babies cry when they are hungry, tired and uncomfortable, in pain or simply when they are bored. Feeding alleviates hunger, but food and drink should not be used to stop other causes of crying or the baby learns to associate all comfort with eating.

- Where possible, babies should be given regular family foods — in appropriate sized portions, chopped or pureed where necessary.

- Try to steer away from special baby foods. They're not necessary and most commercial varieties are so smooth that they encourage the infant to swallow the food quickly without first moving it around much in the mouth.

- Where the main family meal is unsuitable for babies (for example, pies, curries or very spicy foods), either cook some of the basic ingredients without the hot spices or serve a small portion of grilled fish, meat or chicken and some steamed vegetables.

- Fruit is always appropriate for a dessert, peeled, stewed or mashed as needed.

- Let babies feed themselves as early as they are able. Although their first efforts are messy, it helps children learn to eat what and how much they want rather than what someone else efficiently spoons into them.

- Finger foods are a popular choice and even when children can use a spoon or fork, most still like to pick up foods in their fingers. Allow them to enjoy doing this and teach appropriate table manners about which foods it is polite to eat with the fingers when they are old enough to understand such niceties.

Young children

When children go to pre-school and then school, they're subjected to peer group pressure to choose particular foods, or even particular brands of foods. Television is also a major influence. Once children begin to watch television, they see many advertisements, almost all of which promote foods of low nutritional value. These have a persuasive effect and encourage children to pester their parents or carers to buy certain foods — generally those with added colourings, artificial flavourings and a high content of sugar, fat or salt. Children need proportionately more nutrients than adults to allow for growth, but they have no instinctive way of choosing the foods they need for good nutrition.

STRATEGIES FOR PARENTS

- Junk foods need not be forbidden, but the quantity most children consume needs to be reduced.

- Divide foods into 'everyday' foods and 'sometimes' foods. Children can grasp this concept from an early age.

- Set a good example with your own eating and drinking habits.

- Eat together as a family as often as possible rather than encouraging children to snack frequently.

- Take children shopping for fruits and vegetables.

- Involve children in cooking foods from scratch and give them responsibility for preparing some meals for the family, for example, Saturday lunch.

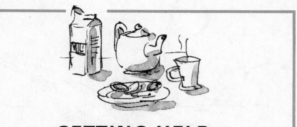

GETTING HELP

For those children who are overweight, it is best to change their diet and exercise patterns as soon as possible. A health professional seeking to help an overweight child will generally want to know the child's current food habits, general state of health and how the child's environment affects his or her food habits. Routine eating habits give a clue to the foods and drinks the child eats in appropriate quantities, which ones are omitted and where there may be some overindulgence. A dietitian or doctor can analyse a child's eating habits and give appropriate advice, but parents and teachers can also play a role.

STRATEGIES FOR SCHOOLS

- Ask a local doctor or dietitian to come and talk to parents, students and school canteen staff.

- Switch to a healthy canteen (this is now mandatory in some states).

- Join a School Canteen Association and enrol in one of the healthy canteen competitions.

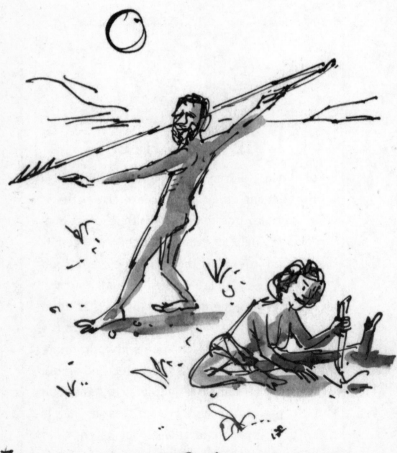

LEAN HUNTER GATHERERS ...

Adolescents

When adolescents reach their period of peak growth, they are usually ravenous. Growth requires a high level of nutrients and kilojoules. Those who also play a lot of sport may have an amazing appetite, consuming huge meals and wanting more within a couple of hours. This is normal but unfortunately, many hungry teenagers satisfy their hunger with junk foods and develop poor eating habits.

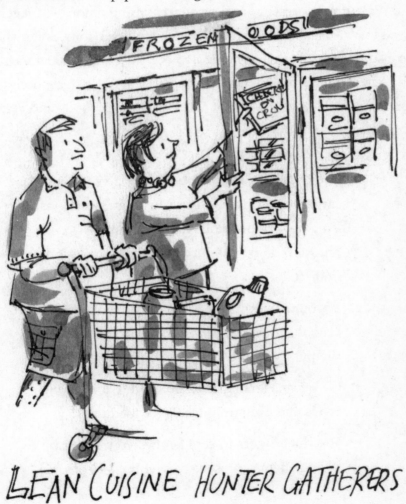

LEAN CUISINE HUNTER GATHERERS

Some teenage boys continue to eat as though they are growing rapidly even after their growth rate slows. If this also coincides with a period of lower physical activity — which may accompany studying or spending more time watching sport than actually participating — excess body fat accumulates. This is the current pattern in many communities, with obesity climbing rapidly. In Australia, 32% of 16–18 year-old boys and 27% of girls are overweight or obese.

Peer group pressure is particularly strong among teenagers and this also leads to poor eating and drinking habits. Soft drink consumption is high and many do not realise that a 600 mL bottle of soft drink contains the equivalent of about 16 teaspoons of sugar. A high consumption of fast foods, snack foods and alcohol also causes problems.

STRATEGIES FOR PARENTS

- Satisfy your child's appetite by giving them larger portions of nutritious foods such as breads, cereals and grains, meat, fish or chicken, dairy products (preferably low fat) and fruits.

- Encourage teenagers to exert pressure on their school canteen if it is still selling junk foods (help is available from state governments).

- Give teenagers more responsibility for buying foods and preparing meals for the family.

- Teach teenagers to cook, either yourself or by giving them a present of say, Italian cooking lessons.

What is a balanced diet?

So what food and nutrients do children need? The human body is an efficient machine and like any machine, needs energy to function. We get energy from food and it can be measured in kilojoules (kJ) or kilocalories (commonly written as Cals).

A balanced diet contains all the essential nutrients in approximately the amounts needed for healthy living, to contribute to well being and maintain health. The essential nutrients include proteins, fats, carbohydrates, vitamins, minerals, dietary fibre and water. Natural plant chemicals, called phytonutrients, may also be important for long-term health. No one food contains all the nutrients in the amounts the body needs, so we need to choose a variety of fresh natural foods.

Proteins

The body normally uses all the protein in the diet for growth and daily repair of tissues. Some can also be burned as a source of energy. Protein is not usually converted to body fat. Each gram of protein contributes 17 kJ of energy.

Protein is found principally in animal foods like meat, fish, chicken, eggs and dairy products (milk, cheese and yoghurt) but also in plant foods such as legumes, various beans, including soya beans (from which tofu is made), and nuts and grains (including pasta and cereals). Fruit and vegetables have very little protein.

Fats

Fats exist as saturated or unsaturated fatty acids. The foods listed below contain essential unsaturated fatty acids that are important for the structure of membranes around all body cells. Essential fats also have a vital role in the brain and nervous system and protect the body against inflammatory reactions. All fats supply high levels of energy with each gram having 29 kJ and excess energy from fats is easily converted to body fat.

Foods that contain essential fats include:

- fish;

- nuts;

- wholegrains;

- seeds, especially sunflower, pumpkin (pepitas), sesame or linseed;

- vegetable oils (olive, sesame, sunflower, canola).

Carbohydrates

Carbohydrates are important sources of readily available energy. They are found with other important nutrients in foods such as the ones listed below. Sugar is also a source of carbohydrate, but contains no other needed nutrients so should play only a minor role as a source of carbohydrate. In practice, most people can only eat excessive quantities of carbohydrate in the form of sugar or when the carbohydrate is accompanied by fat.

There is great debate about whether excess carbohydrate is converted to body fat. Early studies suggested that excess carbohydrate increased the amount of energy the body used and that very little was converted to fat. More recent research suggests that some people can convert carbohydrate to fat more easily than others. However, in all cases, if the body is busy burning carbohydrates as a source of energy, it may not get around to burning fat and any fat eaten is then deposited as body fat.

The best carbohydrates are those that come with other nutrients and are slowly converted to blood glucose — known as having a low glycaemic index (GI). A low GI on its own is not a mark of a 'good' carbohydrate as some fatty foods and highly processed snacks or desserts may have a low GI even though they lack essential nutrients and can create dental decay.

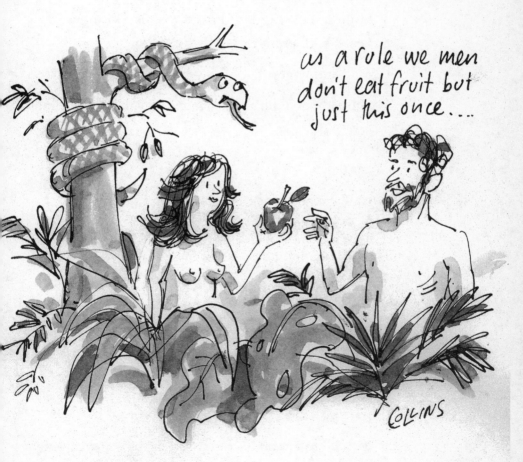

Carbohydrates are found with other important nutrients in:

- fruit;

- potatoes;

- breads;

- grains and cereals (breakfast cereals, pasta, rice, wheat, buckwheat);

- legumes such as soy beans (used to make tofu or soy beverages), chick peas (used in hoummus), canned baked beans, kidney beans and lentils;

- milk and yoghurt.

Foods with carbohydrate but no other useful nutrients include:

- soft drinks;

- cordials;

- confectionery such as jelly beans, 'snakes' or barley sugar.

Foods with carbohydrate plus fat include:

- bread with a spread;

- pasta with a fatty meat or creamy sauce;

- fried rice;

- potatoes with sour cream or butter;

- potato chips.

Foods with large quantities of fat as well as some carbohydrate include:

- chocolate;

- cakes;

- biscuits;

- crisps and similar snack foods;

- pastries;

- ice cream;

- many desserts.

Nutritionists classify such foods as fatty foods rather than carbohydrate foods. Some low carbohydrate diets damn all carbohydrates, although it would make more sense if they reserved their censure for carbohydrate foods that are also high in fat.

Vitamins

Vitamins are needed for the maintenance of all normal bodily functions. There are 13 different vitamins, each with a distinct function in the body that cannot be fulfilled by any other nutrient. They are found in a range of foods, including fruits, vegetables, meat, fish, chicken, eggs, dairy products, breads, cereals, grains, seeds, nuts and some vegetable oils. Vitamin supplements are not required unless a child has allergies or some other reason for avoiding a range of regular foods.

- **Vitamin A** exists in a ready-made form (also called retinol) in milk, cheese and eggs or as beta carotene in brightly coloured fruits and vegetables. The body converts beta carotene to vitamin A.

- **Vitamin B** consists of 8 separate vitamins: thiamine (B1), riboflavin (B2), niacin (B3), pantothenic acid (sometimes called B5), pyridoxine (B6), folate, biotin and cyanocobalamin (B12). The B vitamins are found in wholegrain products, vegetables, meat, fish, legumes, yeast extracts and dairy products. The B vitamins most likely to be lacking in children and adolescents in Western countries are folate and vitamin B12. Folate is found in green leafy vegetables, avocado, oranges, breads and breakfast cereals with added folate, beetroot and salmon. Vitamin B12 is found only in animal foods, but is also added to some soy products.

- **Vitamin C** is found in fruits (including juices) and vegetables. Supplements of vitamin C are popular but unnecessary and their acidity makes them a dental hazard, especially if taken in the form of chewable tablets. There is no evidence to justify giving children vitamin C to help prevent colds.

- **Vitamin D** comes mainly from the action of sunlight on the skin. A total exposure time for some portion of the skin for 1–2 hours a week supplies enough. It is also found in fatty fish such as herrings and sardines and is added to some brands of margarine.

- **Vitamin E** is found in nuts, wheatgerm, seeds (such as pumpkin and sunflower) and the oils made from seeds and nuts, peanut butter, wholegrains and vegetables.

- **Vitamin K** comes mostly from synthesis in the intestine. It is also present in green leafy vegetables, mushrooms and cauliflower.

Minerals

Among the many minerals needed, the most likely to be present in short supply are **calcium** and **iron**. Calcium is found in dairy products (milk, yoghurt and cheese), calcium-fortified soy beverages, almonds, fish and other seafood and some green vegetables. A form of iron that is well absorbed (haem iron) is found in meat, chicken and fish. Non-haem iron is less well absorbed but helps to make up the total iron levels. It is found in wholegrain and fortified cereals, wholemeal bread, green vegetables, legumes and eggs.

Fibre

Dietary fibre is also important to keep the intestine healthy and prevent constipation. It is found only in plant-based foods, with the highest quantities in wholegrain cereals and breads, legumes, fruits and vegetables.

Water

Water is even more vital to life than food and is needed for every bodily process. The best source of water is — water! Although this may sound trite, it's true. Soft drink manufacturers claim that their products are important as sources of water, but if you get your water from soft drinks, you also get highly acidic ingredients that damage tooth enamel (especially in regular or diet cola drinks) plus a lot of sugar (or artificial sweeteners), preservatives, artificial colourings and flavourings. There is no need for breast-fed infants to be given water, but after 6 months of age, children can (and will) drink water happily, as long as they are not introduced to sweetened cordials and juices. Older children will also drink water, although advertising of other drinks makes them popular too. For everyday use, water is the desirable beverage for children.

Healthy eating guidelines

Like many countries, Australia has established a set of dietary guidelines for children and adolescents, which are general principles to apply from birth to 18 years of age.

- Encourage and support breastfeeding.

- Children need appropriate food and physical activity to grow and develop normally. Growth should be checked regularly.

- Enjoy a wide variety of nutritious foods.

- Eat plenty of breads and cereals, vegetables (including legumes) and fruits.

- Low-fat diets are not suitable for young children. For older children, a diet low in fat and in particular, low in saturated fat, is appropriate.

- Encourage water as a drink. Alcohol is not recommended for children.

- Eat only a moderate amount of sugars and foods containing added sugars.

- Choose low-salt foods.

There are also guidelines on specific nutrients.

- Eat foods containing calcium.

- Eat foods containing iron.

In translating these guidelines into a variety of foods to enjoy every day, the best approach is to choose foods from each of the five food groups every day. These are:

- breads, cereals, rice and pasta;

- vegetables and legumes (various beans);

- fruit;

- milk, yoghurt and cheese;

- meat, fish, poultry, eggs, nuts, legumes;

The appropriate quantities of foods from these groups will vary with age, appetite and activity level, but try to achieve these proportions in your children's meals:

- **plenty of** plant foods, breads, cereals, rice, pasta, vegetables, legumes and fruits;

- **moderate amounts of** animal foods (milk, yoghurt, cheese, meat, fish, poultry, eggs);

- **small amounts of** extras such as oils and other fats;

- **no** alcohol.

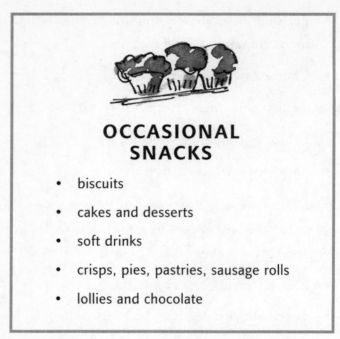

OCCASIONAL SNACKS

- biscuits

- cakes and desserts

- soft drinks

- crisps, pies, pastries, sausage rolls

- lollies and chocolate

STRATEGIES FOR PARENTS

Here are some ways to encourage children to eat foods from the five food groups, and to encourage variety.

Breads and cereals

- Start infants on smooth wholemeal bread or wholemeal toast fingers.

- If toddlers and school-aged children only want white bread, buy a high-fibre white loaf or a sour-dough bread.

- Gradually move children from baby porridge to rolled oats or healthy cereals like Weetbix or Vita Brits.

- Use fruit loaf or fruit buns.

- Make French toast using raisin bread (use fat-reduced milk in the egg–milk mixture).

- Explain to school-aged children that highly sugared breakfast cereals are a rip-off because they get you addicted to sugar and cost more even though sugar is less expensive to food companies than the basic cereal grains.

- When giving children spaghetti, noodles and rice, avoid adding fatty or salty sauces and serve them as meals rather than for snacks.

- Make damper on an outside fire (when weather conditions permit).

Vegetables

- Serve raw carrot sticks, green beans, strips of red and yellow capsicum, cherry tomatoes, celery.

- Let children pick up stir-fried vegetables in their fingers.

- Let children choose vegetables in the supermarket.

- At barbecues, include some small vegetables such as corn-on-the-cob (cut into thirds), baby mushrooms, zucchini and cherry tomatoes on skewers.

- Grow some vegies, such as tomatoes, lettuce (plant each seedling in a pot or large ice cream container), carrots (delicious when small), snow peas or honey-snap peas, green beans.

Fruit

- Leave fresh fruit in a visible spot in the fruit bowl or at the front of the fridge.

- Parents (especially fathers, who may not normally eat much fruit) can set a good example by eating more fruit.

- Choose appropriate-sized pieces of fruit — small apples or apple slices are best for small children.

- Teach children (and adults) to taste different flavours by buying several varieties of apples, slicing them and comparing their flavours.

- If children won't eat fruits like apples or pears because they don't like the skin, peel the fruit for them when eating it at home.

- Cut up fruit for dessert (for example, melon, pawpaw, pineapple).

- Buy mandarins for school lunches as they're easy for little fingers to peel.

Meat, fish, poultry, eggs, nuts, beans, tofu

- Use chicken drumsticks or lamb cutlets so they can be eaten in the fingers.

- If children reject meat because they don't like the idea of killing animals, respect their feelings but point out they need to accept alternative sources of protein such as beans, tofu, peanut butter or eggs.

- Use canned beans, hot or cold.

- Mash tofu and avocado together as a spread for toast or bread.

- Use smooth peanut butter in a saté sauce to serve with crisp raw vegetables.

Dairy products

- If children don't want to drink milk, make sure they get their daily allowance by using it on cereal, in custard or junket instead.

- Substitute yoghurt for milk, if desired.

- Use cheese on pasta, in vegetable pancakes or melted into mashed potatoes, as well as on sandwiches or grilled on toast.

- Make smoothies incorporating milk and yoghurt with fruit and a touch of honey.

- Once children reach 2 years of age, switch to fat-reduced milk.

HEALTHY EATING HINTS

For children who are overweight, the aim is not to put them on a diet, but to encourage the whole family to follow healthy eating guidelines for meals and snacks. A few tips may help.

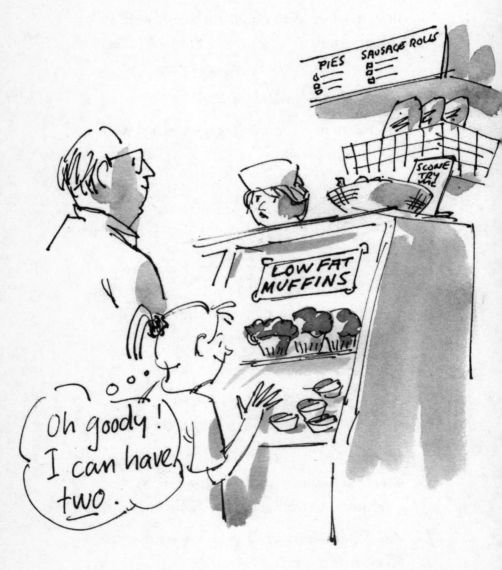

- The whole family needs to follow a healthy eating pattern. Don't expect those who are overweight to eat different foods from other family members.

- Concentrate on healthy food choices rather than discussing whether a food is fattening.

- Stock the kitchen with healthy foods and don't buy junk foods (soft drinks, lollies, chocolate, biscuits, crisps) as a regular purchase. When children are hungry, they will eat what is available. If only healthy foods like fruit, bread (which can also be used for toast), yoghurt and milk (preferably fat-reduced) are available, that's what children will choose.

- Keep cold water in the fridge, including some in unbreakable bottles so kids can help themselves.

- Respect changes in children's appetites and never insist they finish everything on their plate. This helps no one and can encourage children to ignore their satiety signals.

- Go for quality, where possible. If you buy mushy apples or woody carrots, children won't eat them. Fruits and vegetables in season taste best and are generally cheaper.

- Introduce the idea of menus for different occasions. No child ever goes to McDonald's and asks for pizza because they know it's not

on the menu. Even young children can understand the concept that you have everyday
foods, party foods, holiday foods and feast
foods. And just as they accept they can't wear
party clothes to school, so they quickly accept
that party foods are not for everyday use.

- Make a few rules and stick to them. Most parents have rules about bed time for younger children and which television programs they can
watch. Snacks and meals need a few rules too.
One rule might be that crisps, lollies and biscuits aren't suitable for the school lunchbox.

- Make special fruits treat foods — for example,
a few strawberries, cherries or other stone fruits
(in season), lychees, sliced mango or melon.

- Serve foods such as noodles as part of a main
meal rather than using them as snacks.

- Try to eat together as a family rather than having each person get themselves a quick meal.

- Eat at the table, not in front of the television.
When we eat while doing something else (like
watching television), we are often unaware of
what we are eating.

- Break the habit of eating in the car. If you're
going on a long journey, stop to have something to eat rather than nibbling as you go.
During short trips, children do not need to eat.

Why three meals a day?

We eat three meals a day because it's a pattern that fits in with our body's needs for fuel. Most meals take about 5 hours to be digested, and this coincides with times of feeling genuine hunger pangs. Growing children need extra food and many will use up the fuel from a meal before the next one is due. In such cases, healthy snacks can fill the gap, but it is important not to establish a habit of snacking on foods with poor nutritional quality.

Breakfast

Almost all babies wake up and want to be fed. But between infancy and starting school, about 10% of children pick up poor habits and go off to school without eating a meal that provides energy to kick-start their day. The situation doesn't improve, and 15% of teenagers skip breakfast.

Many studies show the body functions best when we break our overnight fast with a healthy breakfast. Research has tended to concentrate on the effects breakfast has on children's performance, with most studies showing this valuable meal improves various aspects of brain function. The results are usually most dramatic in children who are less well nourished but even among those who have more than enough food, researchers have shown that breakfast eaters make fewer mistakes and work faster in arithmetic tests. One Danish study also found higher ratings on tests of creativity and physical endurance in children who ate breakfast.

Fewer studies have concentrated solely on adults' breakfast habits but there are reports that when subjects eat breakfast, they have better recall of visual images and words than when they skip this important meal. There is also some limited evidence of higher rates of accidents among those who drive or operate machinery after skipping a meal. Similar findings may be relevant in children but studies have not yet extended to young people. There's no mystery to the better results in most studies of breakfast eaters — laboratory results clearly show more favourable blood glucose levels in those who eat regular meals, especially if the meals contain carbohydrates.

Many school teachers say they don't need formal studies because a lack of attentiveness during the late morning hours is a dead giveaway as to which children haven't eaten breakfast!

Over the last 20 years, many studies have shown that overweight people are more likely to skip breakfast than those within the healthy weight range. The data have been collected from research in the United States, Japan, France, the United Kingdom and Spain and have included children, teenagers and older adults.

Even though research shows clearly that eating breakfast is associated with a lower BMI, skipping this important meal is becoming more common throughout the developed world — parallelling the spread of obesity. There's no way eating breakfast could solve the problem of obesity, but it is at least a possible contributing factor that is easy to fix.

A BALANCED BREAKFAST

The important nutritional components of a good breakfast include:

- fluid to replace losses from the lungs during the night;

- some type of carbohydrate such as fruit, cereal, bread, rice, milk or yoghurt to replenish blood sugar levels, which decrease during the night;

- some type of fruit (or vegetable) to provide nutrients, including vitamin C, which then helps the body absorb more iron from other foods.

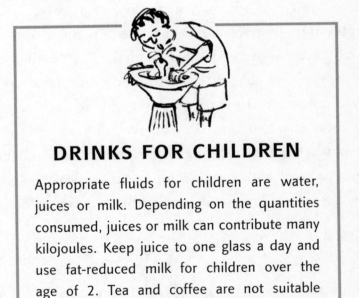

DRINKS FOR CHILDREN

Appropriate fluids for children are water, juices or milk. Depending on the quantities consumed, juices or milk can contribute many kilojoules. Keep juice to one glass a day and use fat-reduced milk for children over the age of 2. Tea and coffee are not suitable for young children but are fine, in moderation (2–4 cups/day), for teenagers.

The Glycaemic Index

Carbohydrate foods are broken down to blood glucose at varying rates. Foods that are converted to glucose slowly have a low glycaemic index (GI) and may be more suitable for anyone who needs to lose weight as they delay the return of hunger. The GI is a valuable tool to add to other methods of choosing foods, but should not replace basic choices made on the basis of a food's nutrients. It is only ever suitable to use within a food group. It is valid to choose a low GI wholegrain or sour dough bread over a white loaf but such choices should not be extended to selecting chocolate rather than bread just because chocolate has a low GI. Some advertisements distort the principles of the GI with statements such as 'ice cream has a lower GI than carrots', implying ice cream may be a better choice than a carrot. Always choose foods first on the basis of their overall nutritional value, and then use the GI to decide within a food category. However, remember that the overall GI of a meal is based on averaging values for foods within that meal. Potatoes may have a relatively high GI but if eaten in a meal with a low GI food such as peas, the overall GI value becomes moderate and perfectly acceptable.

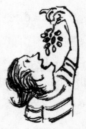

So far, the only evidence that choosing low GI foods helps with weight loss has come from very small short-term studies. Most studies show advantages if people with diabetes make low GI choices, but no effect on weight. Suitable healthy breakfast foods with a low GI include:

- rolled oats;

- natural muesli;

- sultana bran or other high fibre cereals;

- most fruit (especially apples, oranges, pears, grapes, kiwi fruit, berries and stone fruits);

- wholegrain or sourdough breads or toast;

- baked beans.

ADD AN EGG

Growing children need plenty of protein and many find breakfast more satisfying if they have an egg, although cereals, breads and dairy products (including fat-reduced varieties) also provide protein. Bacon and fried eggs are too fatty to eat often, but a boiled or poached egg has many more pluses than minuses and can be happily added to a child's breakfast. Eggs contain cholesterol, but most excess cholesterol occurs when the body is stimulated to make it from a diet high in saturated fat. An egg has a moderately low level of saturated fat.

Healthy breakfast choices:

- freshly squeezed orange, carrot and celery juice followed by wholegrain toast with a boiled egg;

- smoothie made with low-fat milk, banana, strawberries, yoghurt, honey and wheat-germ and raisin toast;

- a poached egg with grilled mushrooms and tomatoes and a toasted English muffin;

- rolled oats with wheatgerm and dried apricots and toast with yeast extract;

- natural muesli with sliced banana, strawber-ries, melon or peach with fat-reduced milk or soy beverage;

- Weetbix or Vita Brits with milk, followed by multigrain toast with Vegemite and a glass of granny smith apple juice.

SPECIAL OCCASION BREAKFAST

Serve a fruit platter of pawpaw chunks, berries, melon slices, banana and orange segments with fat-reduced honey yoghurt, followed by thin pancakes with a squeeze of orange and lemon juices.

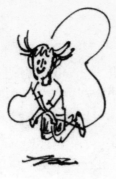

RUNNING LATE?

If children really are regularly too late to eat breakfast, change the time they go to bed and get up. For an occasional time when they are running late, send them off with some fruit and a carton of fat-reduced yoghurt or a soy drink. Breakfast cereal bars are not a good choice because the cereal is held together with a hefty dose of sugar, and in some cases, a helping of unexpected saturated fat. A soy or muesli bar can help out occasionally, but don't make a habit of buying them as most are high in kilojoules and are a dental hazard.

Lunch

There are children who take the same sandwiches for lunch every day from kindergarten to Year 12. Many children like ritual in their meals just as they like order in other aspects of their lives. A seeming lack of variety can be frustrating to parents, but if the foods chosen are basically healthy, it may not matter. At some stage the natural desire to explore other food choices will usually kick in, often at puberty and sometimes only when their peers or a girlfriend or boyfriend exerts some influence. A lack of variety is much more of a problem in young children who will eat only jam sandwiches for lunch or some similar food that doesn't provide the nutrients they need.

By midday, breakfast has been used up by the body and afternoon efficiency depends on a good lunch. Lunch is an important meal and it doesn't make sense to neglect it.

A healthy lunch for children usually consists of sandwiches or rolls plus fruit and a drink. Providing you choose appropriate sandwich fillings, this fairly standard lunch can easily contribute a third of the day's nutrients for most children. Skip the spread or use light cream cheese or avocado mixed with lemon juice (which stops it going brown). As children grow, simply increase the quantities of sandwiches and add extra fruit. Avoid adding packeted snacks to the lunchbox.

When parents work outside the home, many children buy their lunch, often purchasing just one roll or sandwich and then filling up on various junk foods. This is unsuitable for all teenagers, whatever their weight, since the meal is unlikely to meet their nutritional needs. Growing active teenagers need more than one sandwich or roll. Whether or not you are busy, encourage teenagers to prepare their own lunch, at least most of the time.

Many families find it easiest to prepare a supply of sandwiches or rolls all at the same time, and freeze them to use for lunch or to supplement freshly made sandwiches on busy mornings. Freezing sandwiches or rolls is especially useful during the hot summer months as the lunch will gradually defrost but will stay cool enough until midday to prevent the growth of undesirable bacteria in meat, chicken, egg or fish sandwiches. Pack some fresh lettuce or tomatoes to add to the sandwiches or bread rolls at lunch time. Pita or various flat breads can also be frozen successfully.

SUITABLE FILLINGS FOR FREEZING

- cold meats
- chicken, or turkey
- most cheeses
- peanut butter
- dried fruit
  (delicious with light cream cheese)
- egg
- sweetcorn
- baked beans
- tuna or salmon

Whether a child takes fresh sandwiches or frozen, it makes sense to freeze a small bottle of water to pack in the lunchbox. The frozen water keeps the sandwiches and fruit cool and will have defrosted by lunchtime to provide a cool drink. If children have not had juice at breakfast, a small juice is also suitable, but if children drink juice every time they are thirsty, their total kilojoule intake can easily increase to high levels.

Many parents pack a 'treat' in the lunchbox — usually a packet of crisps, a cake or muesli bar. These foods are not necessary and contribute a lot of extra fat. Schools are now being encouraged to give guidelines for suitable lunches brought from home and these advise against high fat/high sugar treat foods. These items are best kept for party foods or as occasional treats at home when it is more appropriate to brush teeth after consuming them.

FOR VERY
YOUNG CHILDREN

- Avoid too much choice in the lunchbox. Having to cope with new faces, new subjects, new games and books, young children need a simple lunch that doesn't overwhelm them with choice.

- Cut sandwiches into small triangles and arrange them as they do in sandwich shops so they look attractive and easy to eat.

Healthy lunch choices

- sandwiches made with a choice of bread or rolls (wholemeal, multigrain, rye, white high-fibre, sour dough) plus fillings of salad with avocado, chicken, cottage cheese, fat-reduced cheddar, egg, a slice of lean meat, salmon, tuna or turkey plus a piece of fruit;

- pita bread stuffed with salad and tabbouli or any of the fillings listed above plus a piece of fruit;

- for a change from sandwiches: a cob of corn plus a container of salad vegetables plus some leftover chicken plus a piece of fruit;

- wholewheat or rye crispbread with fat-reduced cheese, a small container of cherry tomatoes and celery plus a piece of fruit;

- lavash bread spread with a mixture of grated carrot, peanut butter and sultanas and rolled into a 'log';

- add an apricot or a peach or plum or a small bunch of grapes or a few strawberries or blueberries, a small new season's apple or some pieces of rockmelon, watermelon or pineapple in a small plastic container.

Dinner

Where possible, try to sit down together as a family for dinner rather than each person getting their own meal and eating it while watching television. When most people watch TV, they are unaware of what they are eating and often don't feel satisfied at the end of the meal. The kinds of foods often eaten in front of television tend to have less emphasis on vegetables and foods that need to be cut up and more on easy-to-eat food such as pastries, pies and pizza.

Dinner for children should contain a good source of protein such as meat, chicken, fish or a vegetarian alternative plus several vegetables (cooked or raw) and a source of carbohydrate such as potato, spaghetti, rice or some other grain. To give an idea of balance, about a quarter of the plate should have meat, half should be vegetables and the other quarter can be the carbohydrate source.

Rich sauces are not suitable for everyday meals and the habit of adding lots of cheese to the top of almost every meal is not recommended. If children want tomato sauce, try to buy one with reduced salt content.

For those who want dessert, offer fresh fruit with yoghurt or fat-reduced ice cream occasionally.

Snacks

Most children get hungry between meals. Those who are very active often find it difficult to sit still long enough at mealtimes to eat enough to last them until the next meal. There is nothing inherently wrong with snacking, providing the snacks make a worthwhile nutritional contribution to the child's daily needs. Most don't.

Healthy snack choices

- fresh fruit: bananas, apples, mandarins, pears, oranges, strawberries, watermelon, rockmelon (or whatever is in season);

- frozen fruit: try peeled bananas, sultana grapes when available, quartered oranges, slices of melon, chunks of pineapple;

- iceblocks home-made from frozen fruit juice;

- fresh bread (most children will peel off a slice and just eat it straight);

- toast or raisin toast;

- toasted muffins;

- wheat or rye crispbread;

- Weetbix or Vita Brits;

- raw carrots;

- banana or other fruit smoothies (use reduced-fat milk, low-fat yoghurt or a small scoop of low-fat ice cream);

- low-fat natural yoghurt blended with frozen berries or canned peaches (these can be frozen in small containers);

- iced water or a pop-top bottle of water.

Fast food

Some people argue that there are no 'good' or 'bad' foods. That is true in that foods don't have any moral value. But it's fair to say that some foods have little nutritional value while others are rich in the nutrients needed for growth and health. When it comes to weight control, avoiding fast food (often called 'junk food') will help progress. Realistically, it's impossible to prevent children eating fast foods forever, so a reasonable compromise might be to restrict fast food to once a week or once a fortnight. One fast food chain in France is currently advertising that patrons should eat their food 'no more than once a week'.

Some fast food chains are introducing healthier choices into their menus, although not all the items included in this category fit such a definition. They may have a lower fat level but they still contribute a large number of kilojoules, often from a high content of sugar. An advertisement boasting that a muffin has less than 10 g of fat does not highlight the fact

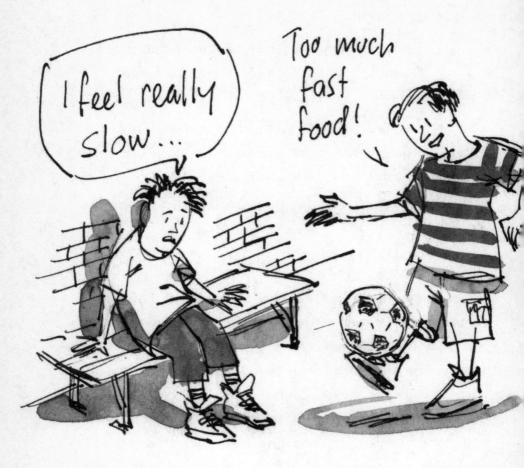

that it contributes a massive 1,600 kJ! Healthier fast food choices are an improvement, and some of the salads are good options, but when most people go to a fast food outlet, they succumb to the allure of the usual fatty offerings.

The healthiest fast food alternatives include grilled seafood, flame-grilled chicken (often available without the fatty skin), kebabs with salad, pizza with half the usual cheese (avoid those with fatty salami) and many Asian meals (but not those in batter or deep-fried).

General tips

- Research shows that those who successfully lose weight and keep it off make breakfast a regular part of their day. Try to set this as a regular family habit.

- Try to identify foods that are healthy as well a being a treat — perhaps strawberries, blueberries, watermelon, prawns, dried peaches, a special bread, frozen yoghurt or low-fat ice cream.

- Rather than serving children heaped plates of food, start with a moderate amount. They may not be hungry enough for seconds, especially if serving dishes are not left on the table.

- Make dessert an occasional extra at the evening meal rather than planning it every night.

- Snack foods are generally high in fat and sugar or salt. Try to stick with fruit most of the time.

- Take care with fat-reduced foods as many companies have replaced the fat with high levels of sugar and the total kilojoule count can still be high. Some people also eat more when the label says 'fat-reduced'.

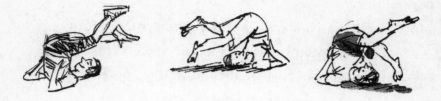

Accepting responsibility

For young children, parents and carers need to take responsibility for making appropriate choices and developing good eating and exercise habits. As they grow older, however, overweight children need to accept that they have to make an effort to monitor their own eating and exercise, although family support will be vital for success. When they're able to accept this responsibility, the key to success is to identify some changes in food and drinks that they can live with and also to find an acceptable and meaningful activity program they can continue with long-term.

It may help to explain to overweight children that everyone has to make greater efforts in some areas of life. For example, some people are naturally good at school work whereas others have to conscientiously try harder. At a more trivial level, some people have hair that just sits the right way; others have to take a bit more effort to make their hair go the way they want it to.

Food labels

Food labels now provide useful information about ingredients and some nutrients. All ingredients must be listed on the label in their order of prominence, with the most abundant ingredient first. The percentage of any ingredient included in the name, or characteristic of the product, must also be stated. For example, an apricot muesli bar would have to list the percentage of apricot present. This helps us know what we're getting for our money and also whether a product is a good buy. For example, if a raspberry fruit drink lists its ingredients as glucose, sucrose, raspberries (2%), colouring, flavouring, preservative, you know that the product is largely made up of the two sugars listed first.

If terms such as 'light' or 'lite' are used, the manufacturer must also explain what the term refers to — light in salt, colour, flavour, fat or whatever. Take care with terms such as 'x% fat-free' as they can be misleading. If minced beef, for example, is marked 80% fat-free, it will have 20% fat, which is a high fat level considering lean meat has about 5% fat. Some products labelled as 98% fat-free may still be high in kilojoules if they contain a lot of sugar. Always check the kilojoule level and compare it with other products rather than relying solely on claims about the fat.

It's also important to check the serving size as this can vary and may be quite different from what you would consume. Consumer information on products such as breakfast cereals and spreads for bread sometimes lists very small serving sizes, presumably to downplay the kilojoule or sugar levels. At other times, the serving size does not seem relevant for the container, as in 200 g tubs of yoghurt where the serving size is listed for a 150 g serve. Studies also show that when a food is labelled as 'low fat', most people take a larger portion.

6

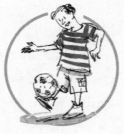

The benefits of exercise

Obesity is a complex condition with interrelated causes. As we have seen, these include over-nutrition, under-activity, a genetic predisposition and a range of social factors. The increased prevalence of obesity in childhood and adolescence means many previously adult health problems are now appearing in children.

Then and now

Past generations did not have the opportunity to be inactive. Throughout history, humans have been physically active in hunting and gathering foods. We evolved as creatures who walked. These days we drive everywhere and children are driven to school, to visit friends, shops and sporting venues.

Even 50 years ago, people were much more active around the home, scrubbing clothes by hand because washing machines were not available, polishing rather than using a spray and wipe solution, pushing a cumbersome lawn mower and using stairs, not lifts and escalators. Children were expected to help with household chores and did not sit watching television or playing on computers until the microwaved or home-delivered meal was ready, as many do now.

There is now a device or machine for almost every piece of physical work required. We change the television channel with a remote control device. Another opens garage doors. We press a button to wind down car windows. We use escalators and lifts instead of stairs and many public buildings do not even have stairs accessible for anything except emergency use. Most important of all, we drive instead of walking — even for short distances — and expect a parking spot within metres of our destination. Cities are designed to give maximum benefits to car drivers rather than pedestrians and many suburbs are now set out with circular streets and no footpaths, assuming that everyone will drive rather than walk.

Suburban housing blocks are also smaller, but new houses are larger, leaving virtually no backyard where children can play. At the same time, development has reduced the amount of public parkland and fear of danger means that many parents will not allow their children to play outside or away from home.

Most people also say they are too busy to walk or don't have time. Small children are strapped into strollers to make things faster for their parents. Initially, the children are unwilling to be confined, preferring to toddle off and explore their surroundings. Soon, however, they become used to the ride and then refuse to walk anywhere.

Changing the way we do things

The components we can change in this situation are food and exercise. If we only change one of these the chance of longer-term success may be relatively limited. However, physical activity and exercise should be the major components of treating obesity in children as they are unrestricted and positive in contrast to restricting food intake, which is passive, restrictive and negative.

Lack of adequate physical activity is one of the prime causes of excess weight in children. Not all inactive children develop a problem with weight, but at any age, failing to use the body causes a decline in health and wellbeing. Regular physical activity is especially essential for normal growth and development in children and for the body to function properly.

Regular exercise builds strength in:

- heart and lungs;
- muscles;
- bones.

Low levels of physical activity, on the other hand, may be directly related to adult health problems such as:

- hypertension;
- cardiovascular diseases;
- obesity.

When people follow diets that restrict kilojoule intake too much, they may appear to lose a lot of weight but this is often accompanied by a loss of protein (from lean body tissue) and a loss of water. By comparison, weight that is lost through exercise minimises the loss of lean tissue. Weight loss without exercise generally results in 25% of the lost weight coming from lean tissue. When appropriate changes in eating habits are combined with exercise, loss of lean tissue is as low as 5%.

BENEFITS OF EXERCISE

- energy expenditure increases
- loss of lean muscle tissue is minimised
- appetite fits more closely with the body's needs
- ill-effects of obesity are minimised
- basal metabolic rate increases

Better eating habits and more exercise can also improve the ratio of lean to fat tissue within the body. When such an improvement does occur, it is possible that it will be accompanied by little or no weight loss in the short term. Occasionally, weight may even increase a little because muscle tissue, which increases with exercise, is dense and heavier than fat tissue. However, even though weight may increase a little in such cases, the body is becoming leaner. The best way to cope with this is not to focus on the scales, but judge progress by how fit the child is and how their clothes look (they should become a little looser).

An activity program is a positive opportunity where the child (and the family) can do something to help themselves. Enjoying exercise on a regular basis can be especially rewarding because it helps improve self-concept and body image. The results of exercise are cumulative and long-term, and improved fitness makes those involved feel good. Exercise also stimulates the body's metabolism for some time after finishing the exercise, so you continue to burn more kilojoules. The length of time the metabolic rate stays higher depends on the intensity and duration of the exercise.

From a young age, we need to establish in children habits of walking and cycling instead of using a car all the time, using stairs rather than escalators and lifts, and watching less television. The best way for parents and carers to do this is to lead by example. As a society, we need to change our attitude to healthy lifestyle habits. There are no magical formulas or products that will take over this role.

All children, irrespective of their age, size and shape, love to move. Sadly, many are not given enough opportunity and encouragement. Quality experiences during childhood and adolescence set the scene for a more active adult life. Key elements in maintaining activity from childhood to adult life are the success, fun and enjoyment we experience in the activities during our younger years. Activity should always be relevant and personally challenging for the individual. Body size and shape play a role in determining physical ability in various activities, so an appreciation of individual differences is important.

Developing movement

Official guidelines for Australian children and adolescents have not been published at the time of writing, but regular physical activity and appropriate eating behaviours should begin at birth.

The first years of life represent an intense period of motor learning that provides the foundation for more complex and skilled activities later. The development of basic movement patterns of crawling, standing, walking, running and jumping is fostered by the opportunity to play. Young children need to explore their environment through movement and experiment with their bodies' movement capabilities. All children want and need to participate in progressively more vigorous and physically challenging activities as they grow.

Movement is vitally important for young children. Some physical activities can be described as 'learning to move' tasks, while others are more 'learning through movement'.

It's called
a stroller
but he never
gets to
stroll...

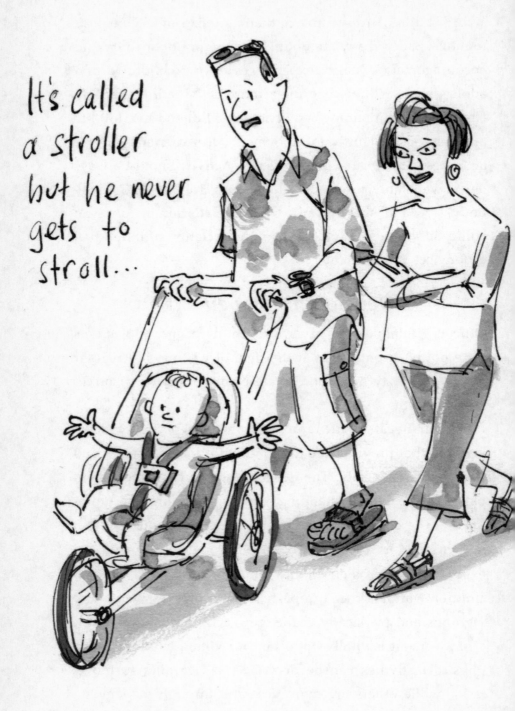

Both types of learning experiences play an important role in children's growth and development. Young children commonly show three different types of physically active play:

1 At first, during infancy, their activity patterns include gross motor movements that appear to have no goal or purpose — for example, kicking their feet or rocking the body. These behaviours occur as babies begin to move major muscle groups as part of their initial exploration. These movements appear to be somewhat random and unplanned and peak about the middle of the first year of life.

2 The second stage occurs at the start of the second year, when children use physically vigorous gross motor movements as they play. This type of play may occur when they are alone or in a social context and it increases from toddler age onwards, peaking at 4–5 years of age and then declining during the primary school years. At about 4 years of age, about one-fifth of children's activity is usually characterised as physically vigorous.

   Early childhood is also a time when socialisation becomes important and behavioural norms are established. This involves a strong dependence on responsible adults, especially during the early childhood years. In their movement tasks, children also rely on their parents or carers as they change from being self-centred to actively seeking assistance. At this stage, children need the approval of others for their physical performance.

3   The third type of physical activity play is rough-and-tumble play and includes vigorous behaviours such as wrestling, kicking and tumbling. This type of play is essentially a social behaviour and usually starts with support from a parent, often the father. A 4-year-old may spend less than 10% of their play time with this vigorous activity, but it usually increases steadily and peaks when children are 8–10 years old.

EVERYONE IS DIFFERENT

Children show individual differences in their growth. They also vary their timing of motor milestones such as crawling and walking. Children also differ greatly in their awareness of the rewards of physical activity — experiences such as self-esteem and self-confidence, and feelings of mastery and competence.

Simple activities can help improve motor skills and simultaneously increase physical activity, although it is always important to match these to a child's stage of development. Children can start with simple games and patterns of physical activity, managing more complex tasks as they move through the various stages of motor development.

First stage

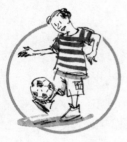

- Provide opportunities for free play with large, soft, lightweight balls.

- Children also enjoy running games, singing games and activities that stimulate their imagination.

Second stage

RUNNING AND DODGING

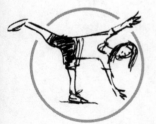

- Join in the fun by chasing children and letting them chase you.

- Set up an obstacle course relevant to a child's age and stage of development. For example, a 3-year-old will enjoy climbing through a hoop tied to the side of a chair, perhaps picking up a child's wheelbarrow and taking it round a tree, jumping over a rope on the ground or walking along a wide plank on the ground.

HITTING

- Hit a ball off the top of a witch's hat or off the ground.

- Try to keep a balloon in the air using either hand.

CATCHING

- Roll a ball between two people.

- Field a rolling ball.

- Catch a large soft ball.

- Catch a small hand-held beanbag with two hands.

THROWING

- Roll a ball underarm, trying to control direction and distance.

- Roll a small ball, concentrating on gripping the ball with the fingers.

- Combine throwing with stopping and catching skills.

BOUNCING

- Combine various tasks with bouncing and catching a large ball.

Third stage

RUNNING AND
DODGING

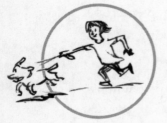

- Include running and dodging tasks with more instructions and extra and more challenging 'obstacles' according to the child's abilities and circumstances.

HITTING

- Bounce a ball and hit or strike with the hand or a bat.

- Hit a ball up against a fence or wall.

- Hit a ball from a stationary position — for example, a T-ball stand.

CATCHING

- Throw and catch overhead.

- Catch a small beanbag with one hand, alternating sides.

- Try two and one-handed catches with various types of balls — for example, small to large.

- Add variety by using two people or a small group to test the same skills above.

KICKING

- Start with a large soft ball.

- Try to kick the stationary ball off the ground. Use alternate feet and gradually add targets and try to kick over a longer distance.

- Think of different soft objects that could be used as balls — for example, empty milk cartons and beanbags.

BOUNCING

- Bounce a large ball with both hands but in different body positions — for example, sitting, kneeling or standing,

- Bounce and catch on the move. Start with walking, then gradually speed up.

- Pat-bounce while walking, then while running.

Fourth stage

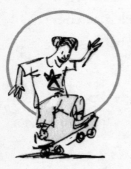

Now your child can move on to more advanced and challenging running and dodging activities. Progressively increase the level of difficulty in: hitting a stationary ball, a ball pitched underarm, hitting a ball to a particular area of the field, hitting tasks using different bats and rackets. Practise more advanced throwing and catching or kicking and catching tasks.

Graded games and games skills encourage body image or body awareness and spatial awareness, as well as eye–hand and eye–foot coordination. All children need activities to develop these skills. Some children will learn more slowly than others. Some, including some larger children, may find simple skills difficult to master at first, but they will be bound to improve with practice and encouragement.

Body awareness

Becoming aware of their bodies helps children develop self-confidence, and a willingness to experiment and understand the body's capabilities so they improve their self-concept. To help children with their body image or body awareness (which includes how they view themselves and their awareness of the relation of one part of the body to another), ask them to try the following:

- touch different parts of the body while standing and sitting;

- move various parts of the body as they are named or get children crawling, moving their arm and leg of one side simultaneously.

Spatial awareness involves children's awareness of their bodies in space and to directions such as up, down, forwards and backwards. As children become more aware of their own body, they can to use various body parts to explore space. Help with this by getting them to move through, in, out, over, around and under various pathways and obstacles.

Eye–hand and eye–foot coordination involves the child's ability to integrate muscles in tasks requiring their eyes and hands or hands and feet. Activities to help include:

- catching and throwing — start with large balls, rolling and bouncing them and gradually moving to smaller balls as the child's abilities improve;

- hitting and striking activities — with bat and ball, racquet and ball, or handball games. Start with simple games such as hitting a stationary ball and progress to hitting a moving ball;

- kicking — start with activities that involve a stationary ball and move to more complex tasks as the child's skill improves.

Be a good role model

If children see their parents sitting around watching television and minimising physical activity, they are likely to pick up the same bad habits. The Australian government recently published National Physical Activity Guidelines for adults advising on the minimum levels of physical activity needed for good health. The guidelines are an excellent starting point for parents who are inactive and who wish to be good role models for their children. For more information about these guidelines, phone 1800 020 103. The guidelines are also available as a brochure and can be downloaded from: http://www.health.gov.au/document/physguide.pdf

The key messages for adults are:

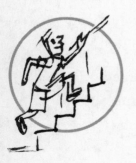

- think of movement as an opportunity, not an inconvenience;

- be active every day in as many ways as you can;

- plan at least 30 minutes of moderate-intensity physical activity on most, preferably all, days (moderate-intensity physical activity will cause a slight, but noticeable increase in breathing and heart rate and may cause light sweating in some people);

- if you can, also enjoy some regular vigorous exercise for extra health and fitness.

Plan enjoyable movement

Just as it is important to eat healthy foods you like, so we all need to find physical activities we enjoy. If your children don't find exercise fun, they won't continue to do it. Everyone's different, but there is bound to be something your child will enjoy: walking, swimming, flying a kite, dancing, bushwalking or birdwatching, riding a tricycle or bicycle and all kinds of sports.

It's a myth that all obese children dislike sport. Although many obese children don't like participating in sport, this is not universal. Many are good at sport and enjoy it. The danger is that some sports have become so competitive that those who show promise are trained and many of the rest give up and become sports spectators. Some children who do not naturally excel at sport prefer not to play at all, for fear of ridicule by their more able classmates.

Many people start playing sport or doing some activity and then drop out. Sometimes this occurs when it all seems too hard. Start children in a sport or activity at a grade where they feel comfortable and competent and match the sport to their interests and abilities as far as possible.

Even more important than specific recreational or sporting pursuits, general activity is important for preventing body fat accumulating. Lack of time is also a classic excuse for not participating in physical activity. A minimal basic level of physical activity should be 'non-negotiable' and people of all ages need to make ordinary activity a part of daily life. We should all aim to be as active as possible rather than always trying to save energy — use the stairs instead of a lift or escalator, for example. Small amounts of activity throughout the day keep the kilojoules burning and all add up to avoid excess weight.

UNSTRUCTURED PLAY

Children who are constantly entertained may lose the skill to explore their environment and play freely. Encourage them to play outside. Research shows that this leads to spontaneous actions and activity that use more energy than occurs with most formal play programs where children spend much of their time standing around waiting for their turn.

Walking

Young children love to go for a walk. They can be slow, but it is time well spent and adults can also learn to re-experience the delight of a child's curiosity and ability to notice features of the everyday environment that we otherwise miss because we take it for granted. If it's not safe for your children to walk alone, go with them.

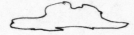

Jack and Jill
were driven
up the hill ...

- Avoid using a stroller — at least some of the time — and let toddlers walk.

- Go bushwalking with your children. Get some details about birds in your area from the local council or the nearest National Parks office. See how many birds you can spot.

- Walk your dog or borrow one from a neighbour regularly.

- Set up a 'walking bus' in your neighbourhood. It works like this: a group of parents decide to walk with their children to school. The one furthest away starts the 'bus' and walks to the house of the next child where that parent takes over and guides the 'bus' to the next house, and so on until the children reach the school. See: www.walktoschool.info

Strategies for schools

- Encourage children to be active by making plenty of play areas available.

- Encourage children to walk to school.

- Arrange activity sessions during morning recess, lunch and after school (where appropriate).

- Explore opportunities to increase physical activity within subject areas such as Maths or Geography.

Other ideas for increasing physical activity

- Make a family rule when you're going out that if the distance to be travelled is less than, say 2 kilometres, you will walk or ride bikes (if appropriate) rather than drive.

- Play backyard cricket. If you don't have a backyard, organise a game at the nearest park.

- Visit the beach or a local swimming pool. Build sandcastles at the beach.

- Arrange lessons for kids (and adults, if appropriate) in tennis, squash, golf or whatever sport the family enjoys.

- Fly kites.

- Dance — inside if the weather is bad or outside if it's fine.

- Play ball games.

- Buy kids active toys or sports equipment for birthdays (kites, balls, a cricket bat, tennis racquet, badminton set or bike).

- Take active holidays at the beach or go camping, skiing, bushwalking or canoeing.

- Encourage the kids to make a garden and grow some vegetables. If you don't have space, try pot plant gardening, using ice cream containers or pots.

- Start a chart with stars for how many days each family member goes for a swim, a bike ride or some other relevant activity.

- Look for opportunities for safe active play.

- Provide children with the opportunity to experience as wide a range of fun activities as possible.

- Involve as many family members as possible in enjoyable activities.

- Give children defined and appropriate active tasks around the home.

TV RULES

- Do not buy a television for any child's bedroom.
- Limit television times for the whole family.
- Negotiate with children that they can watch television after an agreed amount of physical activity.

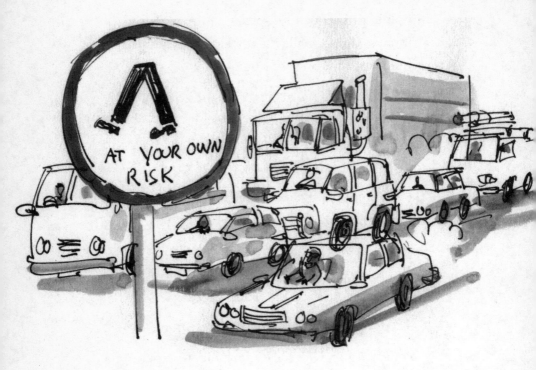

AT YOUR OWN RISK

Encouragement and praise

Parents should encourage physical activity from birth by providing the right opportunities and ensuring that young children's physical activity experiences are positive and fun. The early years are the best time to capitalise on the spontaneity and sheer pleasure that young children get from being active. It may be easier to sit a child in front of the television and some parents discourage physical activity because it leads to more mess and a less tidy house, but it is important to encourage children's natural desire for active play. Support children in anything that increases their physical activity. Encourage children to practise and reinforce movement skills, joining in at least sometimes.

If we want to encourage a lifetime of physical activity, each child also needs to experience some success in their physical activity. Those who have poor physical activity experiences in childhood tend to participate less in physical activity later in life. This is one way that weight problems can develop and be perpetuated. So remember to praise children's efforts and join in their fun as they master different physical activities. Not all children will end up with equal sporting ability, but all children can be good at some physical activity, even if it's simply achieving the ability to enjoy a good walk.

Many children are not given the opportunity to be active enough to establish a sound motor skill base during their growing years. Fundamental movement skills act as a 'tool kit' to develop more complex skills. A good level of motor skill is essential to broaden physical activity opportunities. However, this should not be confused with a high level of proficiency. A level of competency in the activity domain is one of the factors likely to have a bearing upon participation levels in later years, either in team sports or individual types of physical activity that don't involve competition.

Guidelines for physical activity

The main messages for physical activity have been summarised by the National Association for Sport and Physical Education (NASPE) in the United States:

For infants

- Include daily dedicated activities that help them explore their environment.

- Ensure safe settings that facilitate physical activity and do not restrict movement for prolonged periods of time.

- Encourage physical activities that help them develop movement skills.

- Ensure their environment meets or exceeds recommended safety standards so they can enjoy large muscle activities.

- Be aware of the importance of physical activity and facilitate the child's movement skills.

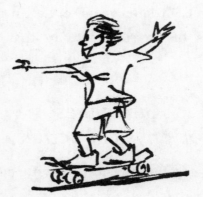

For toddlers and pre-schoolers

Children's ability to move freely and confidently and engage in fundamental movements such as running, jumping, throwing and catching do not occur by chance — children need opportunity, encouragement and support to develop these skills.

- For toddlers, aim to accumulate at least 30 minutes daily of structured physical activity. For pre-schoolers, aim for at least 60 minutes.

- Allow at least 60 minutes and up to several hours each day for daily, unstructured physical activity and avoid sedentary behaviour for more than 60 minutes at a time, except when sleeping.

- For toddlers, develop movement skills that are building blocks for more complex movement tasks. For pre-schoolers, develop competence in movement skills that are building blocks for more complex movement tasks.

- Ensure indoor and outdoor areas meet or exceed recommended safety standards for large muscle activities.

- Be aware that physical activity is important to facilitate children's movement skills.

7

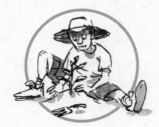

The bigger picture

Prevention is the key

With the rapid rise in overweight and obesity throughout the world, we can no longer sit back and assume that no action is needed to prevent weight problems. If we continue to eat so much and choose so many foods of poor nutritional value while minimising physical activity, the problem will continue to grow. Since overweight children have a high chance of becoming overweight adults, preventing obesity in children should be a high priority for governments, health professionals, families and schools. Physical activity should be a non-negotiable component of our lifestyle from birth, and parents, teachers, sports coaches, doctors and other adults have a collective responsibility to provide every opportunity for young people to be physically active. Making healthy changes is therefore needed throughout the community — not just in those families where someone is overweight.

The role of the school

Schools, especially primary schools, provide an ideal opportunity for intervention and prevention of overweight and obesity. Involvement from parents and other family members add value to school-based health and physical education programs, which should be designed to have something relevant for participation by all children.

The three Rs are important, but so is physical health, so sport should not be seen as an 'extra', but as a vital part of the curriculum from kindergarten to Year 12. The school setting

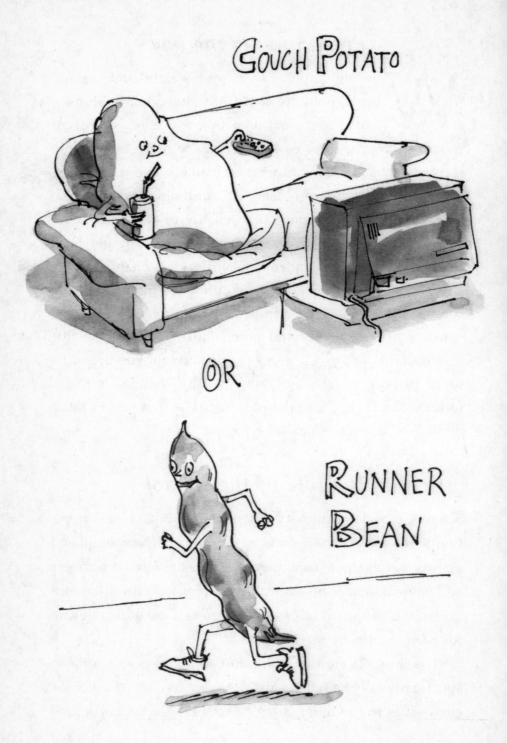

can foster active behaviour in infant, primary and secondary schools. Activities should cater for all children, not just those who are physically capable in the traditional competitive sports. Bushwalking, orienteering, canoeing, building and maintaining gardens (including making compost) or bush regeneration may appeal to children who do not like the usual sports offered.

We fail as a society if we do not provide opportunities for quality activity in the school and community, including safe places for children to walk, play or ride their bicycles. Childhood is the best time to teach the next generation about physical activity and healthier eating habits and introducing strategies to maximise participation levels would be a great investment in the health status of future generations. Short-term decisions by governments tend to overlook such long-term benefits.

The school canteen

All schools teach children about nutrition — unwittingly in many cases. Either they teach them that healthy eating is important or, by neglecting the subject and setting a bad example in the school canteen, they give out a strong message that good nutrition is not important. Schools therefore need to establish a nutrition policy that encompasses the school canteen. Teachers cannot teach healthy eating in the classroom if the canteen is selling a different story.

If your school canteen sells junk foods to children, try to influence it to change. Most schools rely on canteen profits. Many therefore condone selling children junk foods on the basis that it is helping the school. It may be helping finances, but this policy is certainly not helping the children's future health.

School canteens are small businesses and their profit depends on how efficiently they are run. Some schools selling only healthy foods make a handsome profit and some that sell heaps of junk food have low profit levels. Any owner of a successful small business will confirm that you should never sell your main product at a loss. The major influence on profits is the price of the main sellers — sandwiches and rolls. Some schools sell these at or below cost, and then use junk food sales to make up profit levels.

Children themselves often expect the canteen to sell only healthy foods. Of course, they may *like* the fact that they can buy junk foods, just as they would be happy if the library was stocked with comics and cartoons or junk movies dominated the school's video collection. But they don't *expect* the school to sell junk foods, any more than they expect it to sell cigarettes. They see schools as places that are supposed to set a good example.

Where schools have made the change to a healthy canteen, the children have been the easiest people to convince. A few teachers have objected to their favourite cakes not being available for morning tea, but it is parents who have generally raised the strongest objections. Those who want unhealthy foods sold fear that profits will fall without them and many see nothing wrong with the junk foods that are a regular part of their diet at home. Some take the attitude that 'a little bit of what they fancy won't hurt them'.

Not all parents think like this. Some are incensed that they have brought their children up to eat healthy foods and then have their good example destroyed by the school canteen.

To improve foods in schools:

- check if your state government has rules about what foods can be sold (these are being developed);

- get the principal on side;

- set a desired profit level for the canteen and ask a parent who is an accountant to advise on appropriate selling prices of major selling lines to make that profit;

- invite the local dentist and a dietitian to a parents' meeting to discuss the canteen's food choices;

- contact the school canteen association in your state for lists of approved products and suggestions;

- suggest small changes gradually. For example, canteens could sell hot popcorn instead of potato crisps on some days, provide frozen fruits instead of cakes and switch from pies to hot cheese rolls (made by placing a slice of cheese into a bread roll and heating the roll in the pie oven until the cheese melts and the roll is crisp).

- healthy foods take longer to prepare than packet items and school canteens may need more flexible rosters that do not require the same person to work on the same day every week or month. Ask unemployed people to help out in the school canteen. If they work well, the school can give them a valuable reference for work well done;

- encourage the canteen to advertise products with an eye-catching specials board outside the canteen.

Sports coaches

Children and teenagers should not have to endure unnecessary pressure to be ultra skinny. Sports coaches, for example, should not constantly push girls of normal weight to become thinner. They should also keep an eye out for athletic boys who may also become obsessed with extreme leanness, usually exercising excessively rather than eating little. Parents and sports coaches need to understand that rapid weight-loss is unhealthy for everyone, but especially for growing children and teenagers.

Local community issues

Town planning influences physical activity. Most suburbs and regional areas are now designed on the assumption that car travel is the normal mode of transport. Footpaths may be absent and public transport is often non-existent or unreliable. Large centralised shopping centres (with parking) mean that few people walk to the shops.

Economic advancement and increasing population density lead to many challenges to society, including sufficient areas and facilities for recreation. We need streets that are safe for walking, with well-lit footpaths and cycle ways. Working through local councils as well as state and federal governments, communities can encourage more physical activity with changes to the physical environment. Town planning should include parks and sporting facilities and allow people to walk or catch public transport rather than having to drive everywhere.

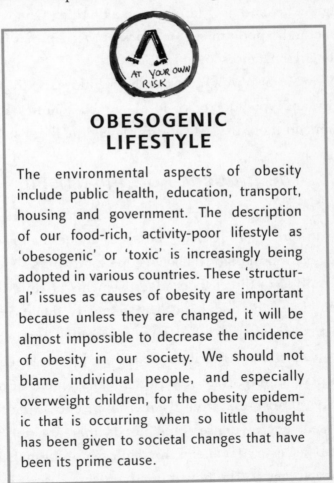

AT YOUR OWN RISK

OBESOGENIC LIFESTYLE

The environmental aspects of obesity include public health, education, transport, housing and government. The description of our food-rich, activity-poor lifestyle as 'obesogenic' or 'toxic' is increasingly being adopted in various countries. These 'structural' issues as causes of obesity are important because unless they are changed, it will be almost impossible to decrease the incidence of obesity in our society. We should not blame individual people, and especially overweight children, for the obesity epidemic that is occurring when so little thought has been given to societal changes that have been its prime cause.

The role of health professionals

If you are concerned about your child's weight, the first person to contact is your family doctor. Ideally, he or she will keep a record of each patient's height and weight and can compare this with desirable levels.

Often, a doctor can suggest simple changes to daily diet and physical activity, which may be all you need. In some cases, however, doctors do not have the time to go into enough detail and may recommend a dietitian who will have long enough appointments to work out a plan that fits your family circumstances and needs.

There are also programs that help children with physical activity and your doctor or local council should be able to recommend those that use appropriately qualified staff.

The influence of advertising

Food advertising on television promotes an unbalanced diet and is in direct conflict with messages about healthy eating. Many health professionals believe manufacturers should not be permitted to direct food advertisements at children who are too young to understand the persuasive intent of advertisements. If junk food ads were not permitted and television programs promoted nutritious foods and physical activity, it could play an important role in the management of obesity. Instead, almost all advertisements promote the highly processed, energy-dense 'junk' foods that are not recommended as everyday items for children's optimal growth and development. The power of advertising is so strong that

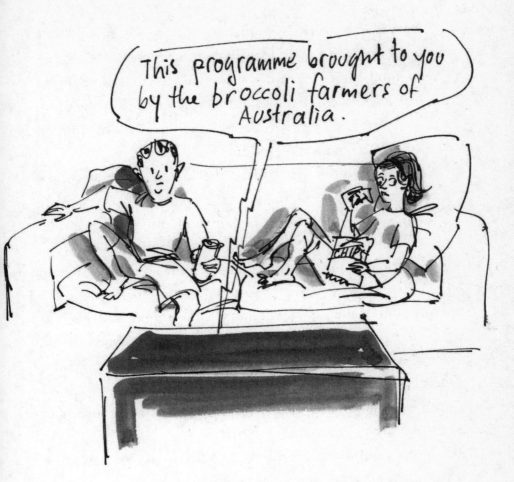

children readily choose products they have seen advertised. This occurs even among 2 and 3-year-olds.

Advertising targets children and, in practice, there are few controls and little policing of these advertisements. In Australia, television stations only have to program 5 hours a week of shows governed by specific guidelines. The standards governing advertisements in children's programs are regularly breached, although the wording of some standards makes this difficult to prove.

Advertising works. Companies would not spend large sums on it if it didn't and studies confirm its effects on children's food choices. There is also evidence that after seeing advertisements, children pester their parents to buy the product advertised. Even when parents say 'no', 80% of children continue to demand the product.

Research shows that up to the age of 4, children see advertisements as entertainment. By age 6–7, they believe advertising is there to provide them with information and up to 8 years of age, children do not distinguish between information and intent to persuade. Some studies show that around 10–12 years of age, most children can understand the motives and aims of advertising. Others find that even at this age, the majority cannot give an explanation of television advertising that shows they understand sales techniques. Older children also believe advertising is a promise of superior quality and value it as a source of information to guide their purchases.

In this context of children's inability to develop a critical attitude towards advertising, food advertising is particularly problematic, since the majority of television advertisements are for foods or drinks that are high in saturated fat, sugar or salt. There are no advertisements for carrots, for example.

There are various ways to help children overcome the effects of advertising. These include:

- joining the push from many health professionals to lobby politicians to ban advertising directed at children or when children are the main viewing audience;

- avoiding commercial television (not always practical);

- explaining the persuasive effects of advertising to children;

- resisting children's 'pester power' as much as possible.

The role of government

We need appropriate education programs to alert everyone — whatever their weight — to the facts of obesity. We also need information about what can be done to prevent the occurrence of obesity or reduce its effects. This could help normal-weight children be more empathetic to the plight of those with weight problems and also enhance the self-concept of obese children. Unfortunately, current training for health professionals and teachers does not include adequate information about obesity. Too often, information about obesity and appropriate ways to prevent or correct it is written for commercial gain in the form of the latest diet fad. Instead, we need:

- accurate information about food, physical activity and health to be widely disseminated in the community (including schools and through health professionals);

- effective government policies for school canteens;

- government initiatives to promote cooking and food preparation in all schools;

- effective government curbs on advertising and marketing directed to children;

- local government initiatives to make physical activity safe and available.

Appendix

Sources of information

The Internet

The websites listed here provide extra information in nutrition, physical activity, obesity and related areas. However, be aware that although the Internet can provide useful information, there are also a lot of sites with misleading information.

NUTRITION
- For general information: Nutrition Australia: http://wwwnutritionaustralia.org
- For specific help, contact a dietitian through the Dietitians Association of Australia: http://www.daa.asn.au
- For information on food allergies: The Food Allergy Network: http://foodallergy.org
- If you are suspicious about 'cures', diet products, programs: Quackwatch: http://quackwatch.com

PHYSICAL ACTIVITY
- The Australian Sports Commission aims to increase participation in sports and physical activity among Australians of all ages: Active Australia: http://www.activeaustralia.org
- President's Council on Physical Fitness and Sports: http://www.fitness.gov

- CDC: Nutrition and physical activity: http://www.cdc.gov/nccd-php/dnpa/index.htm
- Health Canada: Healthy Living: http://www.hc-sc.gc.ca/english/lifestyles/index.html
- For lots of activity ideas: http://www.pecentral.org

OBESITY

- Childhood obesity in Australia: http://www.health.nsw.gov.au/obesitysummit and http://dhs.vic.gov.au/phd/obesityforum
- For information about food laws, food additives and food standards in Australia, see http://www.anzfa.gov.au

Supplementary reading

- *The Diet Dilemma Explained*, Rosemary Stanton, Allen & Unwin, Sydney, 2000. Explains and rates different diets and diet products.
- *Healthy Vegetarian Eating*, Rosemary Stanton, Allen & Unwin, 1997. Useful for information for children who don't want to eat meat, discusses vegetarian eating without preaching. Looks at potential advantages and how to avoid potential problems.
- *Growing Up, not Out*, Kate Steinbeck, Simon & Schuster, Sydney, 1998. Written by a well-known endocrinologist as a reliable factual guide for parents.
- *If not Dieting, Then What*, Rick Kausman, Allen & Unwin, Sydney, 1998. Although written for adult women, this book may be helpful for teenage girls who are constantly dieting.
- *When Eating is Everything*, Jillian Ball, Phyllis Butow, Fiona Place, DoubleDay, Australia and New Zealand, 1991. A useful book for girls with eating disorders. Should be available in most libraries.
- *Winning is Kid's Stuff*, Denis Baker, Collins Dove, Victoria, 1988. More appropriate for children who want to take part in organised sports, but includes the idea that sport should be fun. Available in libraries.
- *Kid's Sport: A survival guide for grown-ups*, Denis Baker, Millennium Books, Australia, 1997. Emphasises the fun aspects of children's sport.

- *The Secret of Healthy Children*, Nutrition Australia, Focus Publishing, Sydney, 2003.
- *Food and Play: 2–5 years*, Nutrition Australia, The Australian Nutrition Foundation Inc., 2003.
- *Your Food, Your Body*, Nutrition Australia, The Australian Nutrition Foundation Inc., 2001.

Cookery books with healthy enjoyable recipes

- *Great Food for Men* , Rosemary Stanton, Allen & Unwin, Sydney, 2002. Healthy easy recipes for men to cook. Dad — set a good example!
- *Simply Healthy*, Sally James, JB Fairfax Press, 1999. Great low-fat recipes.
- *Fresh and Healthy*, Sally James, JB Fairfax Press, 2000. More low-fat recipes.
- *Vegetables*, Rosemary Stanton, Allen & Unwin, 2000. An A–Z of vegetables, describing the history of each vegetable plus information on choosing, storing, preparing and cooking them.
- *Rosemary Stanton's Healthy Cooking*, Murdoch Books, Sydney, 1997. Recipes from previous books *Health and Energy* and *Eating for Life*, plus some extra information.
- *The Good Gut Cook Book*, Rosemary Stanton, HarperCollins, Sydney, 1998. Healthy recipes that include fat and fibre counts.

Community contacts

Information is available from baby health centres and child health centres in your state or territory.

Index